T0262987

Myopathies

Guest Editor

ROBERT L. WORTMANN, MD

RHEUMATIC DISEASE CLINICS OF NORTH AMERICA

www.rheumatic.theclinics.com

May 2011 • Volume 37 • Number 2

SAUNDERS an imprint of ELSEVIER, Inc.

W.B. SAUNDERS COMPANY

A Division of Elsevier Inc.

1600 John F. Kennedy Blvd., Suite 1800 ● Philadelphia, PA 19103-2899

http://www.theclinics.com

RHEUMATIC DISEASE CLINICS OF NORTH AMERICA Volume 37, Number 2

May 2011 ISSN 0889-857X, ISBN 13: 978-1-4557-0503-0

Editor: Rachel Glover

Developmental Editor: Eva Kulig

© 2011 Elsevier Inc. All rights reserved.

This journal and the individual contributions contained in it are protected under copyright by Elsevier, and the following terms and conditions apply to their use:

Photocopying

Single photocopies of single articles may be made for personal use as allowed by national copyright laws. Permission of the Publisher and payment of a fee is required for all other photocopying, including multiple or systematic copying, copying for advertising or promotional purposes, resale, and all forms of document delivery. Special rates are available for educational institutions that wish to make photocopies for non-profit educational classroom use. For information on how to seek permission visit www.elsevier.com/permissions or call: (+44) 1865 843830 (UK)/ (+1) 215 239 3804 (USA).

Derivative Works

Subscribers may reproduce tables of contents or prepare lists of articles including abstracts for internal circulation within their institutions. Permission of the Publisher is required for resale or distribution outside the institution. Permission of the Publisher is required for all other derivative works, including compilations and translations (please consult www.elsevier.com/permissions).

Electronic Storage or Usage

Permission of the Publisher is required to store or use electronically any material contained in this journal, including any article or part of an article (please consult www.elsevier.com/permissions). Except as outlined above, no part of this publication may be reproduced, stored in a retrieval system or transmitted in any form or by any means, electronic, mechanical, photocopying, recording or otherwise, without prior written permission of the Publisher.

Notice

No responsibility is assumed by the Publisher for any injury and/or damage to persons or property as a matter of products liability, negligence or otherwise, or from any use or operation of any methods, products, instructions or ideas contained in the material herein. Because of rapid advances in the medical sciences, in particular, independent verification of diagnoses and drug dosages should be made.

Although all advertising material is expected to conform to ethical (medical) standards, inclusion in this publication does not constitute a guarantee or endorsement of the quality or value of such product or of the claims made of it by its manufacturer.

Rheumatic Disease Clinics of North America (ISSN 0889-857X) is published quarterly by Elsevier Inc., 360 Park Avenue South, New York, NY 10010-1710. Months of issue are February, May, August, and November. Business and editorial offices: 1600 John F. Kennedy Boulevard, Suite 1800, Philadelphia, PA 19103-2899. Periodicals postage paid at New York, NY and additional mailing offices. Subscription prices are USD 282.00 per year for US individuals, USD 501.00 per year for US institutions, USD 139.00 per year for US students and residents, USD 333.00 per year for Canadian individuals, USD 619.00 per year for Canadian institutions, USD 395.00 per year for international individuals, USD 619.00 per year for international institutions, and USD 194.00 per year for Canadian and foreign students/residents. To receive student/resident rate, orders must be accompanied by name of affiliated institution, date of term, and the *signature* of program/residency coordinator on institution letterhead. Orders will be billed at individual rate until proof of status received. Foreign air speed delivery is included in all *Clinics* subscription prices. All prices are subject to change without notice. **POSTMASTER:** Send address changes to *Rheumatic Disease Clinics of North America,* Elsevier Health Sciences Division, Subscription Customer Service, 3251 Riverport Lane, Maryland Heights, MO 63043. **Customer Service: 1-800-654-2452 (US and Canada). From outside of the US and Canada: 314-447-8871. Fax: 314-447-8029. For print support, e-mail: JournalsCustomerService-usa@elsevier.com. For online support, e-mail: JournalsOnline Support-usa@elsevier.com.**

Reprints. For copies of 100 or more of articles in this publication, please contact the Commercial Reprints Department, Elsevier Inc., 360 Park Avenue South, New York, New York, 10010-1710; Tel.: (+1) 212-633-3813, Fax: (+1) 212-462-1935, and E-mail: reprints@elsevier.com.

Rheumatic Disease Clinics of North America is covered in *MEDLINE/PubMed (Index Medicus), Current Contents/Clinical Medicine, Science Citation Index, ISI/BIOMED,* and *EMBASE/Excerpta Medica.*

Printed and bound by CPI Group (UK) Ltd, Croydon, CR0 4YY

Transferred to Digital Print 2011

Contributors

GUEST EDITOR

ROBERT L. WORTMANN, MD, FACP, MACR
Professor of Medicine, Section of Rheumatology, Department of Medicine, Dartmouth Medical School and Dartmouth Hitchcock Medical Center, Lebanon, New Hampshire

AUTHORS

ALAN N. BAER, MD
Associate Professor of Medicine, Division of Rheumatology, Johns Hopkins University School of Medicine, Good Samaritan Hospital, Baltimore, Maryland

STEVEN K. BAKER, MSc, MD, FRCP(C)
Associate Professor, Department of Medicine, McMaster University, Hamilton, Ontario, Canada

LISA CHRISTOPHER-STINE, MD, MPH
Assistant Professor of Medicine and Neurology, Division of Rheumatology, Department of Medicine, Johns Hopkins University School of Medicine, Baltimore, Maryland

JEFFREY A. COHEN, MD
Professor of Neurology, Dartmouth Medical School, Hanover, New Hampshire; Section Chief of Neurology, Dartmouth Hitchcock Medical Center, Lebanon, New Hampshire

AREEG EL-GHARBAWY, MD
Biochemical Genetics Fellow, Division of Medical Genetics, Department of Pediatrics, Duke University Medical Center, Durham, North Carolina

ANDREW GOMEZ-VARGAS, MD, PhD
Neurology Resident, Department of Medicine, McMaster University, Hamilton, Ontario, Canada

DOUGLAS W. GOODWIN, MD
Associate Professor of Radiology and Orthopaedic Surgery, Dartmouth Medical School; Director of Musculoskeletal Imaging, Department of Radiology, Dartmouth-Hitchcock Medical Center, Lebanon, New Hampshire

BRENT T. HARRIS, MD, PhD
Associate Professor, Director of Neuropathology, Departments of Pathology and Neurology, Georgetown University Medical Center, Georgetown University, Washington, DC

SABIHA KHAN, MD
Rheumatology Fellow, Division of Rheumatology, Department of Medicine, Johns Hopkins University School of Medicine, Baltimore, Maryland

DWIGHT D. KOEBERL, MD, PhD
Associate Professor, Division of Medical Genetics, Department of Pediatrics, Duke University Medical Center, Durham, North Carolina

INGRID E. LUNDBERG, MD, PhD
Professor of Rheumatology, Rheumatology Unit, Department of Medicine, Karolinska University Hospital, Karolinska Institutet, Solna, Stockholm, Sweden

MATTHEW C. LYNCH, MD
Neurophysiology Fellow, Department of Neurology, Dartmouth Hitchcock Medical Center, Lebanon, New Hampshire

HAL J. MITNICK, MD
Professor of Medicine, Division of Rheumatology, Department of Medicine, New York University School of Medicine, New York, New York

CARRIE A. MOHILA, MD, PhD
Neuropathology Fellow, Division of Neuropathology, Department of Pathology, University of Virginia Health System, Charlottesville, Virginia

ADAM MOR, MD
Resident, Division of Rheumatology, Department of Medicine, New York University School of Medicine, New York, New York

KANNEBOYINA NAGARAJU, DVM, PhD
Associate Professor of Integrative Systems Biology and Pediatrics, Department of Integrative Systems Biology, Research Center for Genetic Medicine, Children's National Medical Center, The George Washington University Medical Center, Washington, DC

LAWRENCE H. PHILLIPS II, MD
T.R. Johns Professor and Vice-Chairman of Neurology, Department of Neurology, University of Virginia School of Medicine, Charlottesville, Virginia

MICHAEL H. PILLINGER, MD
Associate Professor of Medicine and Pharmacology, Division of Rheumatology, Department of Medicine, New York University School of Medicine, New York, New York

DIANNA QUAN, MD
Associate Professor of Neurology, Director, Electromyography Laboratory, Department of Neurology, University of Colorado Denver, Aurora, Colorado

EDWARD C. SMITH, MD
Assistant Professor, Division of Pediatric Neurology, Department of Pediatrics, Duke University Medical Center, Durham, North Carolina

GUILLERMO E. SOLORZANO, MD
Assistant Professor, Department of Neurology, University of Virginia School of Medicine, Charlottesville, Virginia

ROBERT L. WORTMANN, MD, FACP, MACR
Professor of Medicine, Section of Rheumatology, Department of Medicine, Dartmouth Medical School and Dartmouth Hitchcock Medical Center, Lebanon, New Hampshire

Contents

> Idiopathic inflammatory myopathies are a heterogeneous group of autoimmune disorders predominantly affecting skeletal muscles, resulting in muscle inflammation and weakness. The 3 most common inflammatory myopathies are polymyositis (PM), dermatomyositis (DM), and inclusion body myositis. This review details the clinical findings noted in PM, DM, and the emerging entity of autoimmune necrotizing myopathy.

> Recent advances have increased the understanding of the pathogenesis of polymyositis and dermatomyositis. Clearly, the pathogenesis is complex, and adaptive (eg, autoimmune) and innate and nonimmune pathways play a role in the disease mechanisms, but the relative contribution may vary between patients and in different phases of the disease. Phenotyping patients using autoantibody profiling has resulted in information on molecular pathways that may be relevant in certain subsets of patients with polymyositis or dermatomyositis, but combining the autoantibody profiles with molecular signatures of innate and nonimmune mechanisms would enhance our ability to classify, diagnose, and treat these disorders more effectively.

> Inclusion body myositis (IBM) is the most common acquired myopathy in people older than 50 years. IBM typically presents with distal upper extremity weakness accompanied by proximal lower extremity muscle weakness. Associated clinical findings include asymmetric weakness, foot drop, and dysphagia. The pathogenesis of IBM is not clear. In this article the authors briefly discuss postulated pathogenic mechanisms. Although no proven pharmacotherapy exists, some promising candidates are discussed.

> In paraneoplastic muscle disease, the malignancy may remotely affect neuromuscular transmission or incite muscle inflammation or necrosis. In several of these diseases, an autoimmune basis for the muscle disease

has been established and has become a defining feature. These paraneo-plastic muscle diseases may be the first manifestation of a malignancy, and their diagnosis thus demands a vigilant search for an underlying tumor. This article is focused on inflammatory and necrotizing myopathies and disorders of neuromuscular transmission that may arise in the setting of malignancy and are considered paraneoplastic phenomena.

describes how magnetic resonance images are formed and how the signal intensities in T1- and T2-weighted images may be used for diagnosis of the above-mentioned conditions and injuries.

Matthew C. Lynch and Jeffrey A. Cohen

Electromyography and nerve conduction studies are the primary electro-diagnostic studies employed in the evaluation of patients with weakness and suspected myopathy. This article discusses the physiologic principles that serve as a framework for understanding the purpose, limitations, and interpretation of these tests. In the process the authors also review the differential diagnosis of myopathy.

Andrew Gomez-Vargas and Steven K. Baker

Neuromuscular diseases (NMD) constitute a group of phenotypically and genetically heterogeneous disorders, characterized by (progressive) weakness and atrophy of proximal and/or distal muscles. The objective of molecular testing is to confirm the pathogenicity of a relevant sequence variation by correlating an individual's phenotype with what is expected in a given condition. Within the last two decades the application of molecular genetic strategies has led to a delineation of subgroups of clinically indistinguishable NMDs and has disclosed marked disease overlap. The expanding number of molecular defined NMDs requires new strategies to classify overlapping and clinical indistinguishable phenotypes.

Brent T. Harris and Carrie A. Mohila

This review introduces/refreshes some basic histopathologic methods and findings of skeletal muscle biopsies with emphasis on those diseases commonly encountered in a rheumatologist's practice. The 3 general areas of myopathology discussed are metabolic myopathies, toxic myopathies, and inflammatory myopathies. The authors, neuropathologists, hope to provide in this article what they think are some commonalities and disease-specific methods in their pathologic workup, as well as a practical approach to the collaboration that pathologists undertake with their rheumatology colleagues to come to a working diagnosis.

THE CLINICS ARE NOW AVAILABLE ONLINE!

Access your subscription at:
www.theclinics.com

Preface

Myopathies

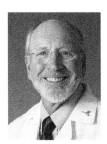

Robert L. Wortmann, MD, MACR
Guest Editor

Diseases that affect skeletal muscle often pose diagnostic problems for clinicians for several reasons. First, the myopathic symptoms are limited to fixed weakness, exercise intolerance, and myalgias (aches, cramps, and pains that may or may not be related to exertion). Whereas fixed weakness portends a pathologic cause, exercise intolerance and myalgia are experienced by everyone at some time or other. Many times it is challenging to differentiate those symptoms due to pathology versus those related to our personal expectations or what we ask of our body.

In addition, the tests we use to diagnose muscle diseases are generally nonspecific. The serum creatinine kinase, the enzyme typically considered to be a marker of muscle disease, can be elevated in some asymptomatic individuals or result from exercise, trauma, or use of various drugs. On the other hand, levels may also be normal in patients with some myopathies. Electromyography too often shows no abnormalities or nonspecific changes. And the range of changes seen on muscle histology is limited. Indeed, muscle biopsy results are rarely diagnostic.

Finally, there are few clinicians that consider themselves myologists. A patient with a suspected myopathy may be referred to a rheumatologist, neurologist, geneticist, or physiatrist. Although each of these specialtists has "some muscle" in their curriculum, none of them cover the area in a comprehensive fashion. It is likely that most clinicians evaluating patients with myopathic symptoms feel somewhat insecure unless the diagnosis is obvious. Furthermore, anyone who is practicing mycology has some formal training but a lot of self-learning has gone into their development. So their confidence may actually be somewhat lacking as well.

With regards to rheumatologists, most are well versed in the evaluation and treatment of the inflammatory myopathies. How much that has to do with the fact that Bohan and Peter, who put order into the classification of these diseases, trained in rheumatology is uncertain. It is more likely that myositis can be seen in patients with other rheumatic diseases such as systemic lupus erythematosus, scleroderma, and mixed connective tissue disease.

Rheum Dis Clin N Am 37 (2011) ix–x
doi:10.1016/j.rdc.2011.02.001
0889-857X/11/$ – see front matter © 2011 Elsevier Inc. All rights reserved.
rheumatic.theclinics.com

In 1975 Bohan and Peter did a remarkable job of taking a field that was in total disarray and providing some order.[1] The scheme they proposed for the classification of polymyositis[1] (which we would now call the idiopathic inflammatory myopathies) continues to be used today despite never having been validated. They proposed that the findings of proximal muscle weakness, nonsuppurative inflammation on muscle histology, elevated levels or serum enzymes derived from skeletal muscle, and a classic triad of changes on electromyography could be used to identify patients. The patients identified then could be further classified as having polymyositis, dermatomyoisitis, myositis with a malignancy, childhood dermatomyositis, and overlap syndromes (subsequently inclusion body myositis has been added to the list). The application of these criteria can be credited with greatly improving research in the field and better treatments for patients.

Another important, but often overlooked, feature of their work was their recognition that "there are certain findings, herein called exclusions, whose presence should make one very cautious about rendering the diagnosis of polymyositis or dermatomyositis." The list of exclusions included central or peripheral neurologic diseases, muscular dystrophy, sarcoidosis, infections, certain drugs and toxins, rhabdomyolysis, metabolic myopathies, endocrine disorders, myasthenia gravis, and other unusual conditions. Therefore Bohan and Peter used a group of, by themselves, nonspecific findings (criteria) to make a diagnosis of an inflammatory myopathy, but also recognized the "nonspecificity" of the resulting diagnosis because patients with many other diseases could fulfill the criteria.

One goal of this edition of *Rheumatic Disease Clinics of North America* is to help readers gain a better understanding of the spectrum of diseases of skeletal muscle: not only the diseases that can be identified by applying the Bohan and Peter classification scheme, but also the entities on their list of exclusions. It is also hoped that a review of diagnostic tools available for the evaluation of myopathies will help the reader become a better diagnostician and therefore be able to better help patients with these often puzzling presentations.

Robert L. Wortmann, MD, MACR
Section of Rheumatology
Department of Medicine
Dartmouth Medical School and
Dartmouth Hitchcock Medcial Center
Lebanon, NH 03756, USA

E-mail address:
robert.l.wortmann@hitchcock.org

REFERENCE

1. Bohan A, Peter JB. Polymyositis and dermatomyositis (first of two parts). N Engl J Med 1975;292:344–7.

Polymyositis, Dermatomyositis, and Autoimmune Necrotizing Myopathy: Clinical Features

Sabiha Khan, MD[a], Lisa Christopher-Stine, MD, MPH[b],*

KEYWORDS

- Myositis • Polymyositis • Dermatomyositis
- Inflammatory myopathy

Idiopathic inflammatory myopathies (IIMs) are a heterogeneous group of autoimmune disorders predominantly affecting skeletal muscles, resulting in muscle inflammation and weakness. Along with the musculoskeletal manifestations, involvement of other organ systems is seen, including the skin, cardiac, gastrointestinal, and pulmonary systems. The 3 most common inflammatory myopathies are polymyositis (PM), dermatomyositis (DM), and inclusion body myositis (IBM). Several much rarer syndromes are also described under the broad spectrum of inflammatory myopathies.

This review details the clinical findings noted in PM, DM, and the emerging entity of autoimmune necrotizing myopathy.

The Bohan and Peter[1,2] criteria have been traditionally used to define and diagnose PM and DM. IBM was not part of the original classification but has been included over time. The Bohan and Peter criteria combine clinical, laboratory, and pathologic features to define PM and DM. More recently, newer criteria have been proposed for the classification of myositis but are not yet widely accepted.

EPIDEMIOLOGY

There is a variation in the age at which PM and DM occur. Although DM has a bimodal incidence pattern, peaking during childhood and then again between 50 and 70 years

Funding/Support: Dr Christopher-Stine's work is supported by NIH grant K23-AR-053197.
[a] Division of Rheumatology, Department of Medicine, Johns Hopkins University School of Medicine, 5200 Eastern Avenue, Mason F. Lord Center Tower, Suite 4100, Baltimore, MD 21224, USA
[b] Division of Rheumatology, Department of Medicine, Johns Hopkins University School of Medicine, 5200 Eastern Avenue, Mason F. Lord Center Tower, Suite 4500, Baltimore, MD 21224, USA
* Corresponding author.
E-mail address: lchrist4@jhmi.edu

of age,[3] PM is rare in childhood and occurs mainly after the second decade of life.[4] Both conditions are more common in women. The reported incidence of both PM and DM is 4 to 10 cases per million population per year.[5]

DEFINITION

The most commonly used criteria for the diagnosis and classification of PM and DM are those defined by Bohan and Peter: (1) symmetric proximal muscle weakness; (2) elevation of serum skeletal muscle enzyme levels, including creatine kinase and aldolase; (3) electromyographic (EMG) evidence of the classic pattern of muscular impairment, with polyphasic, short, small motor unit potentials, fibrillation, positive sharp waves, increased insertional irritability, and repetitive high-frequency discharges; (4) muscle biopsy specimens with typical histopathologic findings of degeneration, regeneration, necrosis, and interstitial mononuclear infiltrates; and (5) characteristic cutaneous manifestation of DM, including heliotrope rash or Gottron sign (**Box 1**).[1,2] As mentioned earlier, over time, IBM has been included in these criteria as its own entity.

MUSCULAR MANIFESTATIONS

The classic clinical finding of both PM and DM is the progressive development of symmetric proximal muscle and truncal weakness that develops relatively slowly, over the course of weeks to months. Patients usually report progressive difficulty with everyday tasks requiring the use of proximal muscles, such as rising from a chair, climbing steps, lifting objects, or combing their hair. Fine motor movements that require the use of distal muscles, such as buttoning shirts and writing, are affected only late in the course of the disease, and when found early in the illness, these affected movements should prompt a search for another neuromuscular disorder.[6] Facial muscles remain unaffected; however, pharyngeal and respiratory muscles can become affected, resulting in complications that are discussed in detail later in this review.[6] Often erroneously thought to be painless diseases, both PM and DM may have associated myalgias and muscle tenderness early in the disease course, more often seen in DM.

The exception to this pattern of muscle involvement is amyopathic DM (ADM), in which patients have the classic dermatologic findings of DM without the accompanying muscular findings.[7]

Box 1
The Bohan and Peter classification criteria

1. Symmetric proximal muscle weakness

2. Elevation of skeletal muscle enzyme levels

3. Abnormal EMG results[a]

4. Muscle biopsy abnormalities[b]

5. Typical skin rash of DM[c]

[a] Polyphasic, short, small motor unit potentials; fibrillation; positive sharp waves; insertional irritability; and bizarre, high-frequency, repetitive discharges.
[b] Degeneration/regeneration, perifascicular atrophy, necrosis, phagocytosis, fiber size variation, and mononuclear inflammatory infiltrate.
[c] Gottron sign and heliotrope rash.

EXTRAMUSCULAR MANIFESTATIONS

The joints, skin, cardiac and pulmonary systems, and the gastrointestinal tract are affected. Extramuscular organ involvement, such as interstitial lung disease (ILD) and cardiac involvement, is associated with worse prognosis.[8]

JOINT MANIFESTATIONS

Joint involvement can occur in those with PM and DM and is characterized by arthralgias and arthritis. It is usually noted early in the course of disease, involving wrists, knees, and the small joints of the hands. Joint involvement is classically nonerosive and frequently responsive to the treatment of the underlying inflammatory myopathy.[9]

DERMATOLOGIC MANIFESTATIONS

Of the IIMs, 5 have cutaneous manifestations: adult DM, juvenile DM (JDM), DM associated with malignancy, DM with overlap syndrome, and ADM.[10]

Bohan and Peter[2] proposed 5 diagnostic criteria for DM, 4 of which focus on clinical, histopathologic, EMG, and chemical evaluation of muscle inflammation. The presence of cutaneous manifestations is the fifth criterion.

Cutaneous manifestations of DM can precede the onset of myositis by several months, and for up to 2 years. However, it is uncommon for myositis to occur before the onset of cutaneous manifestations. Skin involvement can be the most active component of DM and can be recalcitrant to therapy that is otherwise adequate for treatment of muscle symptoms.[10]

The hallmark cutaneous manifestations of DM can be divided into 5 categories: pathognomonic, highly characteristic, characteristic, more common in JDM, and rare in DM.[10]

Gottron papules, observed in more than 80% of patients with DM, are considered pathognomonic for DM. They are violaceous flat-topped papules and plaques located over the dorsal aspect of interphalangeal or metacarpophalangeal joints (**Fig. 1E**). Over time, these papules may evolve and develop atrophic, depressed, white centers with prominent telangiectasias.[10,11]

The heliotrope rash, considered highly characteristic of DM, is a periorbital violaceous erythema with or without associated edema of the eyelids and periorbital tissue (see **Fig. 1A**).[11] The rash can become more confluent and involve the entire face.[10]

Characteristic manifestations include Gottron sign, which is a symmetric macular violaceous erythema with or without edema overlying the dorsal aspect of the interphalangeal or metacarpophalangeal joints, olecranon process, patella, and medial malleoli (see **Fig. 1B**).[11] Other characteristic manifestations include macular violaceous erythema in symmetric distribution in classic areas; shawl sign on the nape of the neck, shoulders, and upper back (see **Fig. 1F**); "V sign" on the V-shaped region of the neck and upper chest (see **Fig. 1C**)[12]; and linear extensor erythema involving the extensor aspects of the legs, thighs, arms, fingers, hands, and feet.

Mechanic's hands, also considered characteristic, present with hyperkeratosis, scaling, and horizontal fissuring of the palms and fingers bilaterally. Mechanic's hands can be a manifestation of the antisynthetase syndrome, which is discussed later.[13] This finding is frequently mistaken for contact dermatitis.[10]

Other characteristic findings include nail fold telangiectasias, cuticular overgrowth, and prominent periungual erythema, which are frequently seen in patients with DM (see **Fig. 1D**).[11] Nail fold telangiectasias occur in 30% to 60% of patients early in the course of the illness.[14] Pruritus is a common, but often underrecognized,

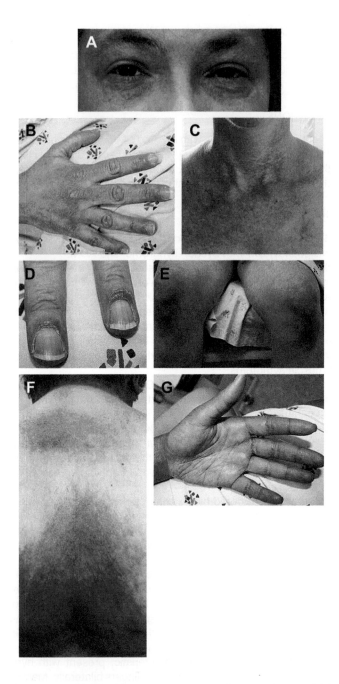

complaint of patients with DM. The presence of pruritus can be helpful in differentiating from cutaneous changes of systemic lupus erythematosus in which pruritus is rare. When cutaneous changes become severe, patients may develop erythroderma, which is total body erythema.[10]

Skin lesions are photosensitive and can be precipitated by both UVA and UVB radiations. A history of severe sunburn preceding the onset of DM has been reported.[4,15]

Cutaneous calcinosis, although more common in JDM, occurring in 30% to 70% of JDM cases, is also seen in adult DM, occurring in 10% of cases.[16,17] It is an often-disabling complication in which subcutaneous calcium deposition occurs in various patterns. Deep deposits occur with linear masses, superficial deposits can erupt through the skin, and reticular subcutaneous deposits can also occur.[13] Cutaneous calcinosis frequently occurs at sites of compression, such as elbows and buttocks, and is associated with increased disease activity and duration. When occurring over the extensor surfaces, cutaneous calcinosis can be painful and can lead to chronic ulceration and infections.[9,16,18]

Rare findings include nonscarring alopecia, erythroderma, vesiculobullous lesions, leukocytoclastic vasculitis, and livedo reticularis. Flagellate erythema has also been noted. It is characterized by erythematous linear lesions on the trunk, back, and proximal extremities and is associated with active disease.[19]

Poikiloderma, a speckled pattern of hypopigmented and hyperpigmented macules interspersed with telangiectasia and cutaneous atrophy on a background of erythema, is a manifestation of disease chronicity that is most commonly found over photo-exposed areas.[20] Severe atrophy of involved skin can lead to fragility, superficial erosions, and ulcerations.[21]

A small subset of patients with DM develop hyperkeratotic follicular erythematous papules that occur in a linear distribution over the dorsal aspect of the hands and feet, frequently over the bony prominences. These papules are known as pityriasis rubra pilaris–like lesions or type Wong DM. The lesions clinically resemble pityriasis rubra pilaris, but they do not have the characteristic findings such as palmoplantar discoloration or desquamating hyperkeratosis. Some of these patients may have concomitant atopic dermatitis.[22]

Cutaneous vasculitis may occur in severe acute forms of DM, with palpable purpura,[23] urticaria-like lesions, livedo reticularis, and digital ulcerations.[24] The presence of leukocytoclastic vasculitis is concerning for an underlying malignancy.[23] Raynaud phenomenon occurs in approximately 25% of patients with DM (see **Fig. 1**G).[25]

ADM

ADM is characterized by the presence of the cutaneous manifestations of DM for 6 months or more in individuals who have normal muscle enzyme levels without evidence of muscle weakness.[26] The term ADM was first coined in 1979 by Pearson,[27] and ADM was eventually recognized as a subset of DM in the 1990s.[28] ADM occurs at an incidence of 9.63 per million persons and represents about 10% to 20% of cases of DM.[29]

◀ ──

Fig. 1. Examples of dermatologic manifestations of DM. (*A*) Heliotrope rash is a very common sign of DM. It can become more confluent and involve the entire face. (*B*) Gottron papules, another characteristic manifestation, are symmetric macular violaceous erythema with or without edema overlying the dorsal aspect of the interphalangeal or metacarpophalangeal joints, olecranon process, patella, and medial malleoli.[11] (*C*) Other characteristic manifestations include the V sign that can occur on the neck and upper chest. (*D*) Image showing cuticular erythema and hypertrophy. Other characteristic findings include nail fold telangiectasias, cuticular overgrowth, and prominent periungual erythema, which are frequently seen in patients with DM.[11] (*E*) Gottron sign, also called Gottron papules, is observed in more than 80% of patients with DM. Gottron papules are violaceous flat-topped papules and plaques located over the dorsal aspect of the interphalangeal or metacarpophalangeal joints. (*F*) Shawl sign, another characteristic manifestation, occurs on the nape of the neck, shoulders, and upper back. (*G*) Raynaud phenomenon occurs in approximately 25% of patients with DM.

Although previously thought less likely, some case studies have suggested that ADM may progress to frank myopathy for up to 10 years after the onset of cutaneous symptoms.[12,29] One study of 16 patients noted that 18.75% of patients developed muscle weakness within 5 years of diagnosis of ADM.[26]

Patients with ADM are at risk for developing the same disease complications as those with DM, such as lung disease and malignancy.[26] The rate of diagnosis of malignancy occurring close to the diagnosis of ADM has been reported between 15% and 28%.[29,30] There have been some reports of the possibility of increased malignancy in ADM compared with DM[30–32]; however, one study of 29 patients with ADM and DM did not find a statistically significant difference between the 2 groups.[29]

CARDIAC MANIFESTATIONS

Cardiac involvement in myositis was first described by Oppenheim[33] in 1899. Historically, it was believed that myositis spared the heart. However, based on autopsy studies, it has become evident that cardiac involvement, although usually asymptomatic, is more common than previously believed.[34] Cardiac involvement is a major cause of mortality in patients with myositis.[34] In a long-term follow-up study, cardiovascular involvement was found to be the most common cause of death in patients with myositis.[8]

The myocardium has been reported to be affected in patients with DM with varying frequencies. Up to 50% of patients with DM evaluated by noninvasive studies have asymptomatic cardiac manifestations.[21,34] Noninvasive studies have shown that up to 85% of patients have abnormal findings on electrocardiography, 77% on ambulatory monitoring, 42% on echocardiography, and 15% on radionuclide ventriculography.[35]

Cardiac manifestations included arrhythmia, conduction abnormalities, cardiac arrest, congestive heart failure (CHF), myocarditis, pericarditis, angina, and secondary fibrosis.[7,8,34]

The frequency of cardiac involvement in myositis has been reported between 6% and 75%.[25,36] Cardiac involvement as a cause of death in PM has been reported between 10% and 20%,[37] although this number is uncertain because large studies are unavailable.

Conduction abnormalities are the most common asymptomatic cardiac manifestation, which are observed in 32% to 72% of patients.[34,36,37] These abnormalities include ST-T changes, bundle branch block, atrioventricular blocks, PR prolongation, Q-wave abnormalities, and arrhythmias. In some cases, patients required pacemaker placement.[25,37]

Arrhythmias and CHF secondary to myocarditis rarely occur in patients with acute disease.[34] In chronic DM, heart failure is seen more frequently and is in fact the most common symptomatic manifestation. The frequency of CHF has been reported to be 3% to 45% in patients with myositis.[37] In chronic DM, heart failure has been attributed to the effects of long-standing hypertension secondary to steroid use.[6] It has also been theorized that the cause of CHF is secondary to myocarditis, leading to left ventricular dysfunction and restrictive cardiomyopathy, or possibly because of fibrosis, resulting in chamber stiffness.[36] It is thought that myocardial involvement resulting in myocarditis occurs by the same mechanism that results in skeletal muscle involvement. Mononuclear inflammatory cells infiltrate into the endomysium and perivascular areas, resulting in degeneration of cardiac myocytes. Histopathologic changes similar to those in the myocardium were also observed in the conduction system, which could explain the cause of heart block.[38]

Angina secondary to Raynaud phenomenon, Prinzmetal angina, and small vessel disease has also been reported in patients with DM.[39]

Pericardial tamponade is very rare, with a frequency reported at about 10%.[25,35,36] However, because tamponade can be fatal, electrocardiography of every case is recommended.[40] Clinically symptomatic cardiac involvement is uncommon, and when present, it is associated with a poor prognosis.[36]

There have also been reported associations between cardiac involvement and anti–signal recognition particle (SRP) antibodies.[13,41] However, more recent evidence suggests that anti-SRP antibodies may not contribute to cardiac involvement to the degree that was once suspected.[42,43]

PULMONARY MANIFESTATIONS

Pulmonary complications are a major cause of morbidity and mortality in patients with PM and DM.[8,44] These complications occur primarily or secondarily due to muscle weakness. Three distinct pulmonary complications of PM and DM have been described: hypoventilation, aspiration pneumonia, and ILD.[45]

Respiratory failure due to hypoventilation has been historically thought to be a rare complication reported in less than 5% of patients with myositis.[46] However, a more recent, larger, retrospective study of patients with DM and PM reported a higher prevalence of 21.8%.[47] Hypoventilation occurs in patients with severe muscle weakness and inflammation, involving respiratory muscles. As a result, restrictive lung function impairment is noted on pulmonary function tests (PFTs). Patients are noted to have reduced lung volumes and maximal inspiratory and expiratory pressures, along with increased residual volumes and normal forced expiratory volume in the first second of expiration (FEV_1) to forced vital capacity (FVC) ratio.[48] Chest radiographs reveal small lung volumes and basal atelectasis.[44]

Aspiration pneumonia is a frequent complication of PM and DM, occurring in approximately 17% of patients.[49] Patients suffering from aspiration pneumonia also frequently complain of dysphagia, which results from disease involvement of the striated muscles of the pharynx and upper esophagus.[44] Aspiration pneumonia is more likely to occur in patients with more extensive muscle and skin disease.[50]

ILD is an inflammatory lung disorder of unknown cause, characterized by infiltrates of monocytes, lymphocytes, and neutrophils, as well as interstitial fibrosis. ILD is a common complication in PM and DM. The incidence of ILD has been reported between 5% and 46% in cross-sectional studies.[44,46,49] No significant difference in the prevalence of ILD exists between patients with PM and DM.[51] ILD associated with myositis may occur before, concomitantly, or after the onset of skin or muscle symptoms.[44,47] ILD associated with ADM is a distinct subset in which the lung disease is rapidly progressive.[44,52]

Myositis-associated ILD occurs in 3 different patterns: (1) acute onset of symptoms, in which patients develop apparent progressive hypoxemia within a month of lung involvement; (2) chronic slowly progressive symptoms; and (3) asymptomatic progression, in which ILD is demonstrated only by abnormal results of chest imaging or PFTs.[51,53]

Cough and dyspnea are the most frequently reported symptoms in ILD, although patients can be asymptomatic. In one study, 27% of patients with ILD were asymptomatic.[54] PFTs demonstrate a restrictive ventilatory impairment and can show decreased total lung capacity, functional residual capacity, residual volume, FEV_1, and FVC, with a normal or elevated FEV_1/FVC ratio and reduced diffusing capacity of lung for carbon monoxide.[44]

Although chest radiography is a useful screening test, high-resolution computed tomography (HRCT) of the lungs is the standard technique for detecting ILD. HRCT is thought to be useful in distinguishing fibrotic disease from active inflammation, with the former presenting as a reticular pattern and the latter as ground-glass pattern.[55]

Bronchoalveolar lavage is not specific for the diagnosis of ILD, although it is useful in differentiating pulmonary symptoms, such as evaluating for infection, drug-induced reaction, and malignancy.[44,56] However, similar to idiopathic pulmonary fibrosis, neutrophil-predominant alveolitis and increased eosinophil counts may indicate more progressive disease.[47] Lung biopsy is not routinely performed for diagnosis because of the increased morbidity associated with the procedure.

Most frequently seen HRCT changes are those of idiopathic nonspecific interstitial pneumonia (NSIP), with irregular linear opacities and with areas of consolidation and ground-glass pattern.[44] However, other patterns such as usual interstitial pneumonia, bronchiolitis obliterans with organizing pneumonia, and diffuse alveolar damage (DAD) are also seen.[44,47]

The presence of antiaminoacyl–transfer RNA (tRNA) synthetase antibodies, of which antihistidyl-tRNA synthetase antibody (anti–Jo-1) is most frequently found, is the strongest predictive marker for ILD.[44] The prevalence of ILD in patients with anti–Jo-1 antibodies is more than 70%.[13,47,54] There are also other markers for ILD, including PM-Scl autoantibodies. Krebs von den Lungen 6, a glycoprotein expressed on type 2 alveolar pneumocytes and bronchiolar epithelial cells, and serum surfactant protein D have been suggested as useful markers for ILD in patients with myositis. However, these markers are not routinely used in clinical practice.[44,57] Serum cytokeratin (CK) 19 fragment, a component of bronchoepithelial cells, is also associated with ILD in myositis. Patients with DAD have higher levels of CK-19 than patients with NSIP.[58]

ILD is considered a major risk factor for premature death. It is unclear if the prognosis of ILD in patients with PM is different from those with DM. However, one study showed that patients with DM-associated ILD were less responsive to steroid therapy than those with PM-associated ILD.[59]

Spontaneous pneumomediastinum has also been reported as a rare complication of myositis-associated ILD, occurring with a prevalence of 8.3% in patients with PM and DM. Pneumomediastinum usually results from rupture of subpleural or paracardial blebs in ILD. In a recent retrospective study, most cases of pneumomediastinum occurred in patients with DM or ADM. Poor survival was associated with an absence of muscle weakness and severe pulmonary involvement before the onset of pneumomediastinum.[60]

Because of the concomitant use of immunosuppressive drugs in the treatment of inflammatory myopathies, infections are another complication to be considered, particularly opportunistic infections. Bronchoalveolar lavage is a useful tool in making the diagnosis.[56]

GASTROINTESTINAL MANIFESTATIONS

Dysphagia to liquids and solids secondary to pharyngeal and esophageal abnormalities has been reported in 32% to 84% of patients with myositis.[61–63] Because of the loss of pharyngoesophageal muscle tone, patients develop nasal speech, hoarseness, nasal regurgitation, and aspiration pneumonia. On examination, tongue weakness, flaccid vocal cords, poor palatal motion, and pooling of secretions can be seen. Proximal esophageal skeletal muscle dysfunction can be seen on manometry with evidence of low-amplitude or no pharyngeal contractions and decreased upper esophageal sphincter pressure.[61]

MUSCLE BIOPSY

A muscle biopsy is required to make a definitive diagnosis of inflammatory myopathy. The biopsy not only confirms the diagnosis but also enables the clinician to rule out other conditions that resemble myositis. It is recommended that a moderately weak muscle is selected for biopsy because it provides the best chance for obtaining information. Because the disease is usually symmetric, the muscle is often best located by EMG testing of the contralateral side (so as not to contaminate the biopsy site with the EMG needle) in combination with magnetic resonance imaging (MRI)-guided biopsy to provide the highest degree of accuracy. An open muscle biopsy is preferred over a needle biopsy because it provides a larger sample.[64]

Characteristic findings of DM are perifascicular atrophy, muscle infarcts, and capillary necrosis with membrane attack complex deposition on vessel walls. Perifascicular atrophy sometimes involves grouped or scattered fibers inside fascicles. It is not uncommon to find punched-out areas of myofibrillar loss that appear as vacuoles at the edge of the fascicle. Muscle fiber necrosis is also seen around the periphery of the fascicle or in a wedgelike distribution suggestive of microinfarcts. Regenerating fibers are also seen. Biopsy results also reveal inflammatory infiltrates in the septa, around vessels, or inside fascicles, although in some instances, inflammation may not be significant. When the inflammation is not significant, the diagnosis hinges on the presence of perifascicular atrophy and reduced capillary density.[64]

Characteristic findings of PM are partial invasion of nonnecrotic muscle fibers by CD8$^+$ cytotoxic T cells and activated macrophages. Also seen is the expression of major histocompatibility complex class I on muscle fiber surfaces, which is not altered by prior immunosuppressive treatment.[64]

LABORATORY TESTING

Laboratory testing reveals an elevation in muscle enzyme levels (CK and aldolase). Extreme elevations in CK levels to of more than 100-fold higher than the upper limit of the reference range are rare in myositis and require evaluation for alternative diagnosis.[7]

ANTIBODIES

The role of antibodies in inflammatory myopathies is unclear. Whether they are involved in pathophysiology or are simply an epiphenomenon is not yet understood.

Autoantibodies to nuclear RNAs and certain cytoplasmic antigens involved in protein synthesis are observed in up to 55% of patients with PM and DM. Anti–Jo-1 antibodies, detected in 20% to 30% of patients with myositis, were the first described autoantibodies in myositis.[13,65] Several strong associations between autoantibodies and clinical phenotypes have been noted. For example, ILD has been observed frequently in patients with anti–Jo-1 autoantibodies.[13]

Antibodies in myositis are categorized into myositis-specific autoantibodies (MSAs) and myositis-associated autoantibodies (MAAs). MSAs are generally found only in patients with inflammatory myositis or in patients with ILD with subclinical myositis, whereas MAAs are also encountered in other connective tissue diseases without signs of myositis (**Table 1**).[13]

Table 1
Autoantibodies in IIM

Antibody	Antigen	Clinical Manifestation
Myositis-specific autoantibodies		
Antisynthetase autoantibodies		
Anti–Jo-1	Histidyl-tRNA synthetase	PM, DM + ILD
Anti–PL-7	Threonyl-tRNA synthetase	PM, DM + ILD
Anti–PL-12	Alanyl-tRNA synthetase	ILD>myositis[a]
Anti-EJ	Glycyl-tRNA synthetase	PM>DM + ILD
Anti-OJ	Isoleucyl-tRNA synthetase	ILD + PM/DM
Anti-KS	Asparaginyl-tRNA synthetase	ILD>myositis[a]
Anti-Zo	Phenylalanyl-tRNA synthetase	ILD + myositis[a]
Anti-Ha	Tyrosyl-tRNA synthetase	ILD + myositis[a]
Nonsynthetase autoantibodies		
Anti-SRP	SRP	Severe, acute, resistant necrotizing myopathy
Anti–Mi-2	DNA helicase	DM with rash > muscle symptoms, treatment responsive
Anti-HMGCR (anti-200/100)	HMGCR	Necrotizing myopathy related to statin use in majority; most patients are statin exposed, but myopathy also reported in a minority of statin-naive patients
Anti-MDA5 (anti–CADM 140)	MDA5	DM: CAM, DM with rapidly progressive lung disease, pneumomediastinum
Anti-155/140	Transcriptional intermediary factor 1γ	CAM
Anti-140	Nuclear matrix protein (NXP-2)	JDM
Anti-SAE	SAE	DM: CAM, DM with rapidly progressive lung disease, pneumomediastinum
Myositis-associated autoantibodies		
PM-Scl	Unidentified	PM or DM/SSc overlap
U1RNP	U1 small RNP	Mixed connective tissue disease (overlap syndrome)
Non-U1 snRNPs	U2, U4/6, U5, U3 snRNPs	PM or DM/SSc or SSc overlap
Ku	DNA-binding proteins	Myositis[a]/SSc/SLE overlap
Ro (SS-A), includes Ro60 and Ro52	RNA protein	Myositis often with SS or SLE, may be associated with ILD (especially Ro52)
56 kDa	RNP particle	Myositis, often with Jo-1
KJ	Unidentified translation factor	PM, ILD, RP
Fer	Elongation factor 1a	Myositis
Mas	tRNA[Ser]-related antigen	Myositis, rhabdomyolysis, chronic hepatitis
MJ	Unidentified nuclear pore	JDM
hPMS1	Protein related to DNA repair	Myositis

Abbreviations: CAM, cancer-associated myositis; HMGCR, HMG-CoA reductase; MDA5, melanoma differentiation–associated gene 5; RNP, ribonucleoprotein; RP, Raynaud phenomenon; SLE, systemic lupus erythematosus; snRNP, small nuclear RNP; SAE, small ubiquitin-like modifier-activating enzyme; SS-A, Sjögren syndrome A; SSc, systemic sclerosis or scleroderma; >, more often than.
[a] May be either PM or DM.

STUDIES/IMAGING

EMG is useful in the diagnosis of myositis and reveals findings in 70% to 90% of patients. Frequent findings include increased spontaneous and insertional activity with fibrillation potentials, positive sharp waves, complex repetitive discharges, early recruitment, and small polyphasic motor unit potentials. Ongoing disease activity is reflected in the amount of spontaneous activity because later in the disease, insertional activity can become decreased because of fibrosis. However, these findings are nonspecific because they can be detected in other muscular diseases.[66]

Along with EMG and muscle biopsy, imaging techniques are important tools in early diagnosis. Imaging studies allow the clinician to determine the extent of disease and also guide biopsy.

Initially, the most important histologic finding at the onset of disease is the presence of inflammatory signs with muscle edema. After an extended period of disease activity, usually in cases that are recalcitrant to therapy, the presence of fat or fibrous tissue changes is detected within muscles. Muscle atrophy is seen after a prolonged disease course but is nonspecific. Although rare, calcification within the muscles can also be seen.[67]

Muscle edema is the most important finding in myositis.[68] Ultrasonography shows increased muscle echogenicity, and fasciae/septa can become obscured with alteration of normal architecture.[67] In a comparison study between patients with IIM and controls, the sensitivity of muscle ultrasonography in detecting myositis was not significantly different from that of EMG or serum CK level analysis.[69] However, ultrasonography offers the possibility of real-time imaging, without exposure to radiation. Doppler imaging in PM and DM reveals hypervascularization and correlates with signs of inflammation on MRI.[70] Ultrasonography is also useful in the detection of subcutaneous calcifications.[71]

Computed tomography (CT) has also been used in the assessment of myositis. CT shows small areas of hypodensity and is useful for detecting fatty infiltration seen in chronic disease. Calcification within the muscles is also more easily detected by CT than MRI.[67]

MRI is more sensitive for the evaluation of muscle edema. The areas of inflammation appear hyperintense on T2-weighted images. Because fat can interfere with the interpretation of MRI images, T2-weighted images with fat suppression or short tau inversion recovery sequences are used to obtain clearer images.[71] Focal areas or diffuse increased signal intensity is a sign of disease activity.[72] The lesions are usually symmetric and prominent in proximal muscles. MRI changes in PM and DM are similar; however, in DM, changes associated with edema are more common than muscle atrophy.[67]

DIFFERENTIAL DIAGNOSIS

When considering the diagnosis of inflammatory myopathy in a patient presenting with muscle weakness, other disease entities must be considered because the clinical presentation may resemble that of myositis.

In patients presenting with early muscle fatigue, elevated muscle enzyme levels, and normal strength, the diagnosis of a metabolic myopathy should be considered. In older patients, the differential diagnosis also includes polymyalgia rheumatica, in which there is proximal muscle stiffness and elevated inflammatory marker levels. However, neither the elevation of muscle enzyme levels nor muscle pathology on biopsy is seen. Polyarteritis limited to muscles has also been reported, in which the patient presents with elevated inflammatory marker levels, myalgias, and slightly elevated muscle enzyme levels.

Another cause to consider is drug-related myopathy, as seen with statins, colchicines, corticosteroids, D-penicillamine, ipecac, cocaine, alcohol, and zidovudine. Hypothyroidism, leading to fatigue, weakness, arthritis, Raynaud phenomenon, and elevated muscle enzyme levels, should also be a consideration. The list of differential diagnoses also includes neuromuscular disorders such as myasthenia gravis and Eaton-Lambert syndrome.[73]

AUTOIMMUNE NECROTIZING MYOPATHY AND THE STATIN CONNECTION

The presence of inflammatory infiltrates in muscle biopsy specimens is a well-recognized feature of autoimmune myopathies. However, muscle biopsy specimens from some patients with autoimmune myopathies contain few, if any, inflammatory cell infiltrates. For example, patients with MSAs directed against components of the SRP have biopsy specimens containing notable for degenerating, necrotic, and regenerating muscle cells without extensive inflammatory cell infiltrates. The authors' group recently tested their hypothesis that patients with otherwise undiagnosed necrotizing myopathies might also have unique autoantibodies that could be used for diagnosis.[74] Among 38 patients with predominantly necrotizing myopathies who underwent muscle biopsy, 12 patients were definitively diagnosed with specific conditions after extensive laboratory testing, who were largely patients with anti-SRP or antisynthetase myositis. The authors screened the sera of the remaining 26 patients for the presence of novel autoantibodies and found that 16 of them immunoprecipitated a pair of proteins with approximate molecular weights of 200 and 100 kDa. The patients with anti–200/100 antibodies did not have other known autoantibodies, including anti-SRP. Thus, anti–200/100 antibodies characterize a unique subset of myopathic patients, representing 62% of the patients with idiopathic necrotizing myopathies.

In many respects, the clinical features of patients with the anti–200/100 antibody immunospecificity are similar to those with other forms of immune-mediated myopathy; the latter typically experienced the subacute onset of proximal muscle weakness with elevated muscle enzyme levels, irritable myopathic findings on EMG, evidence of edema on MRI, and, in most cases, a clear response to immunosuppressive therapy. However, the authors noted several unique features in the patients with anti–200/100 antibodies. First, several patients had very high CK levels (3000–8000 IU/L), with only minimal muscle weakness. Second, in more than 60% of the patients, statin therapy preceded the development of muscle symptoms that persisted despite the cessation of the therapy. Importantly, the authors found that this association was strongest in older patients. Nearly 90% of patients aged 50 years or older who showed positive results for anti-200/100 antibodies had been exposed to statins. In this age-matched comparison, statin use was significantly increased in the patients with anti-200/100 antibodies when compared with patients with DM ($P = .002$), PM ($P = .011$), and IBM ($P = .003$).

Two recent reports described patients who developed necrotizing myopathy with statin use that progressed despite discontinuation of this myotoxic agent.[75,76] In the larger of the 2 series, Grable-Esposito and colleagues[76] described 25 patients who developed an apparently immune-mediated, statin-associated necrotizing myopathy that shares many clinical features with the authors' cohort of patients with anti-200/100 antibodies. For example, these patients had proximal muscle weakness, including men and women in almost equal numbers; had a mean CK level of 8203 IU/L; required multiple immunosuppressive medications to achieve improved strength; and relapsed when immunosuppressive medications were tapered.

SUMMARY

PM and DM are IIMs, each with unique identifying clinical features that reflect differing pathogeneses. Thus, DM is not merely PM plus a rash. Autoimmune necrotizing myopathy is increasingly recognized as a separate category and may have associated primary inflammation, but regeneration, degeneration, and necrosis are the predominant histologic findings. Along with findings of inflammatory muscle involvement resulting in weakness, there are several extramuscular manifestations, including cutaneous (in DM only), cardiac, pulmonary, and gastrointestinal manifestations. Although imaging techniques, EMG, and muscle biopsies allow accurate diagnosis, information obtained from autoantibody testing allows correlation with specific phenotypes. Although studies over the recent years have provided much information about these disease entities, they also reveal that much is yet to be learned.

REFERENCES

1. Bohan A, Peter JB. Polymyositis and dermatomyositis II. N Engl J Med 1975;292: 403–7.
2. Bohan A, Peter JB. Polymyositis and dermatomyositis I. N Engl J Med 1975;292: 344–7.
3. Weitoft T. Occurrence of polymyositis in the country of Gävleborg, Sweden. Scand J Rheumatol 1997;26:104–6.
4. Rider LG, Okada S, Sherry DD, et al. Epidemiological features of environmental exposures associated with illness onset in juvenile idiopathic inflammatory myopathy. Arthritis Rheum 1995;38(Suppl):362.
5. Oddis CV, Conte CG, Steen VD, et al. Incidence of polymyositis-dermatomyositis: a 20-year study of hospital diagnosed cases in Allegheny County, PA 1963–1982. J Rheumatol 1990;17:1329–34.
6. Dalakas M. Polymyositis, dermatomyositis, and inclusion-body myositis. N Engl J Med 1991;325:1487–98.
7. Christopher-Stine L, Plotz P. Adult inflammatory myopathies. Best Pract Res Clin Rheumatol 2004;18:331–44.
8. Danko K, Ponvi A, Constantin T, et al. Long-term survival of patients with idiopathic inflammatory myopathies according to clinical features: a longitudinal study of 162 cases. Medicine (Baltimore) 2004;83(1):35–42.
9. Spiera R, Kagen L. Extramuscular manifestations in idiopathic inflammatory myopathies. Curr Opin Rheumatol 1998;10:556–61.
10. Santmyire-Rosenberger B, Dugan EM. Skin involvement in dermatomyositis. Curr Opin Rheumatol 2003;15(6):714–22.
11. Sontheimer RD, Provost TT. Cutaneous manifestations of rheumatic diseases. 2nd edition. Philadelphia: Lippincott Williams & Wilkins; 2004.
12. Sontheimer RD. Dermatomyositis: an overview of recent progress with emphasis on dermatologic aspects. Dermatol Clin 2002;20:387–408.
13. Love LA, Leff RL, Fraser DD, et al. A new approach to the classification of idiopathic inflammatory myopathy: myositis-specific autoantibodies define useful homogeneous patient groups. Medicine 1991;70:360–74.
14. Kovacs SO, Kovacs SC. Dermatomyositis. J Am Acad Dermatol 1998;39: 899–920.

15. Cheong WK, Hughes GR, Norris PG, et al. Cutaneous photosensitivity in dermatomyositis. Br J Dermatol 1994;131:205–8.
16. Orlow SJ, Watsky KL, Bolognia JL. Skin and bones II. J Am Acad Dermatol 1991; 25:447–62.
17. Dalakas MC, Hohlfeld R. Polymyositis and dermatomyositis. Lancet 2003;362: 971–82.
18. Dasgeb B, Phillips TJ. Adult-onset dermatomyositis complicated by calcinosis cutis. Wounds 2004;16(12):364–70.
19. Nousari HC, Ha VT, Laman SD, et al. Centripetal flagellate erythema: a cutaneous manifestation associated with dermatomyositis. J Rheumatol 1999;26: 692–5.
20. Dugan EM, Huber AM, Miller FW, et al. Photoessay of cutaneous manifestations of the idiopathic inflammatory myopathies. Dermatol Online J 2009;15:2.
21. Miller OF, Newman ED. Dermatomyositis and polymyositis. In: Arndt KA, Leboit PC, Robinson JK, et al, editors. Cutaneous medicine and surgery. Philadelphia: WB Saunders; 1996. p. 283–90.
22. Tribonniere X, Delaporte E, Alfandari S, et al. Dermatomyositis with follicular hyperkeratosis. Dermatology 1995;191:242–4.
23. Feldman D, Hochberg MC, Zizic TM, et al. Cutaneous vasculitis in adult polymyositis/dermatomyositis. J Rheumatol 1983;10:85–9.
24. Yosipovitch G, Feinmesser M, David M. Adult dermatomyositis with livedo reticularis and multiple skin ulcers. J Eur Acad Dermatol Venereol 1998; 11(1):48–50.
25. Hochberg MC, Feldman D, Stevens MB. Adult onset polymyositis/dermatomyositis: an analysis of clinical and laboratory features and survival in 76 patients with a review of the literature. Semin Arthritis Rheum 1986;15(3):168–78.
26. Cao H, Parikh TN, Zheng J. Amyopathic dermatomyositis or dermatomyositis-like skin disease: retrospective review of 16 cases with amyopathic dermatomyositis. Clin Rheumatol 2009;28(8):979–84.
27. Pearson C. Polymyositis and dermatomyositis. In: McCarthy DJ, editor. Arthritis and allied conditions: a textbook of rheumatology. 9th edition. Philadelphia: Lea & Febiger; 1979. p. 742.
28. Euwer R, Sontheimer R. Amyopathic dermatomyositis (dermatomyositis sine myositis). Presentation of six new cases and review of the literature. J Am Acad Dermatol 1991;24:959–66.
29. Bendewald MJ, Wetter DA, Li X, et al. Incidence of dermatomyositis and clinically amyopathic dermatomyositis: a population-based study in Olmsted County, Minnesota. Arch Dermatol 2010;146(1):26–30.
30. Sigurgeirsson B, Lindelöf B, Edhag O, et al. Risk of cancer in patients with dermatomyositis or polymyositis. A population-based study. N Engl J Med 1992; 326(6):363–7.
31. El-Azhary RA, Pakzad SY. Amyopathic dermatomyositis: retrospective review of 37 cases. J Am Acad Dermatol 2002;46(4):560–5.
32. Finger DR, Dunn CL, Gilliland WR, et al. Amyopathic dermatomyositis associated with malignancy. Int J Dermatol 1996;35(9):663–4.
33. Oppenheim H. Zur dermatomyositis. Berl Klin Wochenschr 1899;36:805–7 [in German].
34. Gottdiener JS, Sherber HS, Hawley RJ, et al. Cardiac manifestations in polymyositis. Am J Cardiol 1978;41(7):1141–9.
35. Taylor AJ, Worthman DC, Burge JR, et al. The heart in polymyositis: a prospective evolution of 26 patients. Clin Cardiol 1993;16:802–6.

36. Gonzalez-Lopez L, Gamez-Nava JI, Sanchez L, et al. Cardiac manifestations in dermato-polymyositis. Clin Exp Rheumatol 1996;14(4):373–9.
37. Lundberg IE. The heart in dermatomyositis and polymyositis. Rheumatology 2006;45:iv18–21.
38. Haupt HM, Hutchins GM. The heart and cardiac conduction system in polymyositis-dermatomyositis: a clinicopathologic study of 16 autopsied patients. Am J Cardiol 1982;50(5):998–1006.
39. Riemekasten G, Opitz C, Audring H, et al. Beware of the heart: the multiple picture of cardiac involvement in myositis. Rheumatology 1999;38:1153–7.
40. Chraibi S, Ibnadeljalil H, Habbal R, et al. Pericardial tamponade as the first manifestation of dermatopolymyositis. Ann Med Interne 1998;131:205–8.
41. Targoff IN, Johnson AE, Miller FW. Antibody to signal recognition particle in polymyositis. Arthritis Rheum 1990;33:1361–70.
42. Hengstman GJ, van Engelen BG, Vree Egberts WT, et al. Myositis-specific autoantibodies: overview and recent developments. Curr Opin Rheumatol 2001;13:476–82.
43. Kao AH, Lacomis D, Lucas M, et al. Anti-signal recognition particle autoantibody in patients with and patients without idiopathic inflammatory myopathy. Arthritis Rheum 2004;50(1):209–15.
44. Fathi M, Lundberg IE, Tornling G. Pulmonary complications of polymyositis and dermatomyositis. Semin Respir Crit Care Med 2007;28(4):451–8.
45. Hepper NG, Ferguson RH, Howard FM Jr. Three types of pulmonary involvement in polymyositis. Med Clin North Am 1964;48:1031–42.
46. Dickey BF, Myers AR. Pulmonary disease in polymyositis/dermatomyositis. Semin Arthritis Rheum 1984;14:60–76.
47. Marie J, Hachulla E, Cherin P, et al. Interstitial lung disease in polymyositis and dermatomyositis. Arthritis Rheum 2002;47:614–22.
48. Braun NM, Arora NS, Rochester DF. Respiratory muscle and pulmonary function in polymyositis and other proximal myopathies. Thorax 1983;38:616–23.
49. Marie J, Hachulla E, Cherin P, et al. Opportunistic infections in polymyositis and dermatomyositis. Arthritis Rheum 2005;53:155–65.
50. Medsger TA Jr, Robinson H, Masi AT. Factors affecting survivorship in polymyositis: a life-table study of 124 patients. Arthritis Rheum 1971;14:249–58.
51. Hirakata M, Nagai S. Interstitial lung disease in polymyositis and dermatomyositis. Curr Opin Rheumatol 2000;12:501–8.
52. Suda T, Fujisawa T, Enomoto N, et al. Nonspecific interstitial pneumonia with poor prognosis associated with amyopathic dermatomyositis. Intern Med 2004;43:838–42.
53. Frazier AR, Miller RD. Interstitial pneumonitis in association with polymyositis and dermatomyositis. Chest 1974;65:403–7.
54. Fathi M, Dastmalchi M, Rasmussen E, et al. Interstitial lung disease, a common manifestation of newly diagnosed polymyositis and dermatomyositis. Ann Rheum Dis 2004;63:297–301.
55. Muller NL, Staples CA, Miller RR, et al. Disease activity in idiopathic pulmonary fibrosis: CT and pathologic correlation. Radiology 1987;165:731–4.
56. Ascherman DP. Pulmonary complications of inflammatory myopathy. Curr Rheumatol Rep 2002;4:409–14.
57. Kubo M, Ihn H, Yamane K, et al. Serum KL-6 in adult patients with polymyositis and dermatomyositis. Rheumatology (Oxford) 2003;39:632–6.
58. Fujita J, Dobashi N, Tokuda M, et al. Elevation of cytokeratin 19 fragment in patients with interstitial pneumonia associated with polymyositis/dermatomyositis. J Rheumatol 1999;26:2377–82.

59. Fujisawa T, Suda T, Nakamura Y, et al. Differences in clinical features and prognosis of interstitial lung diseases between polymyositis and dermatomyositis. J Rheumatol 2005;32:58–64.
60. Le Goff B, Cherin P, Cantagrel A, et al. Pneumomediastinum in interstitial lung disease associated with dermatomyositis and polymyositis. Arthritis Rheum 2009;61:108–18.
61. Ebert EC. Review article: the gastrointestinal complications of myositis. Aliment Pharmacol Ther 2010;31(3):359–65.
62. Jacob H, Berkowitz D, McDonald E, et al. The esophageal motility disorder of polymyositis. A prospective study. Arch Intern Med 1983;143:2262–4.
63. de Merieux P, Verity MA, Clements PJ, et al. Esophageal abnormalities and dysphagia in polymyositis and dermatomyositis. Arthritis Rheum 1983;26: 961–8.
64. Dalakas MC. Muscle biopsy findings in inflammatory myopathies. Rheum Dis Clin North Am 2002;28(4):779–98, vi.
65. Nishikai M, Homma M. Circulatory autoantibody against human myoglobin in polymyositis. JAMA 1977;237:1842–4.
66. Briani C, Doria A, Sarzi-Puttini P, et al. Update on idiopathic inflammatory myopathies. Autoimmunity 2006;39(3):161–70.
67. Garcia J. MRI in inflammatory myopathies. Skeletal Radiol 2000;29:425–38.
68. Fleckenstein JL, Reimers CD. Inflammatory myopathies. Radiol Clin North Am 1996;34:427–39.
69. Reimers CD, Fleckenstein JL, Witt TN, et al. Muscular ultrasound in idiopathic inflammatory myopathies of adults. J Neurol Sci 1993;116:82–92.
70. Weber MA, Krix M, Jappe U, et al. Pathologic skeletal muscle perfusion in patients with myositis: detection with quantitative contrast-enhanced US—initial results. Radiology 2006;238:640–9.
71. Walker U. Imaging tools for the clinical assessment of idiopathic inflammatory myositis. Curr Opin Rheumatol 2008;20:656–61.
72. Fraser DD, Frank JA, Dalakas M, et al. Magnetic resonance imaging in the idiopathic inflammatory myopathies. J Rheumatol 1991;18:1693–700.
73. Plotz P. Not myositis: a series of chance encounters. JAMA 1992;268(15):2074–7.
74. Christopher-Stine L, Hong G, Casciola-Rosen LA, et al. A novel autoantibody recognizing 200 and 100 kDa proteins is associated with an immune-mediated necrotizing myopathy. Arthritis Rheum 2010;62(9):2757–66.
75. Needham M, Fabian V, Knezevic W, et al. Progressive myopathy with up-regulation of MHC-I associated with statin therapy. Neuromuscul Disord 2007; 17(2):194–200.
76. Grable-Esposito P, Katzberg HD, Greenberg SA, et al. Immune-mediated necrotizing myopathy associated with statins. Muscle Nerve 2010;41(2):185–90.

Polymyositis and Dermatomyositis: Pathophysiology

Kanneboyina Nagaraju, DVM, PhD[a], Ingrid E. Lundberg, MD, PhD[b],*

KEYWORDS

• Polymyositis • Dermatomyositis • Pathogenesis • Adaptive
• Innate and nonimmune pathways • Skeletal muscle cell death
• Autophagy and endoplasmic reticulum stress

Recent advances clearly have increased the understanding of the pathogenesis of polymyositis and dermatomyositis.[1–8] Immune (adaptive and innate) and nonimmune pathways play a role in the disease pathogenesis. The magnitude and exact nature of the contribution of these pathways to disease initiation and progression are still unclear. Understanding the relative contribution of these pathways is important to design rational therapies for these disorders. Therefore, this review summarizes some of these concepts and recent advances in pathogenic mechanisms in polymyositis and dermatomyositis.

ADAPTIVE IMMUNE MECHANISMS

Inflammatory myopathies are classified as autoimmune diseases because many patients show antibodies to specific autoantigens (eg, anti-Jo) and because of the presence of T cells in large infiltrates in muscle tissue. Another support for the involvement of adaptive immunity is the strong association with HLA-DR genotypes because

Dr Nagaraju is supported by the National Institutes of Health (RO1-AR050478 and 5U54HD053177); Dr Lundberg is supported by the Swedish Research Council, the Swedish Rheumatism Association, King Gustaf V 80 Year Foundation, Funds the Karolinska Institutet, and the European Union Sixth Framework Programme (project AutoCure; LSH-018661) and through the regional agreement on medical training and clinical research (ALF) between Stockholm County Council and Karolinska Institutet. Dr Lundberg has stock ownership in Pfizer, consultancy fee from UCB pharma, and research grant from BMS. Dr Nagaraju has stock ownership in Validus biopharma and consulting fee from BioMarin.
a Research Center for Genetic Medicine, Children's National Medical Center and Department of Integrative Systems Biology, The George Washington University Medical Center, 111 Michigan Avenue NW, Washington, DC 20010, USA
b Rheumatology Unit, Department of Medicine, Karolinska University Hospital, Karolinska Institutet, Solna, SE-171 76 Stockholm, Sweden
* Corresponding author.
E-mail address: Ingrid.Lundberg@ki.se

the function of the HLA-DR molecules is to present antigens to T cells. In addition, the frequent association with other autoimmune and vascular diseases (eg, Hashimoto thyroiditis and scleroderma) coupled with favorable response to immunosuppressive and immunomodulatory therapies in some patients further supports that these myopathies are autoimmune diseases.

Humoral Immune Response

Up to 80% of patients with polymyositis and dermatomyositis have positive antinuclear antibodies and/or specific autoantibodies. Some of these autoantibodies are specific to myositis (eg, aminoacyl transfer RNA [tRNA] synthetases and anti-nuclear helicase [Mi-2]) and others not specific to but associated with myositis (eg, anti-snRNP, anti-Ro/SSA, anti-Ku, and anti-PMS1). Some of these antibodies are clearly associated with distinct clinical features of the disease; for example, anti-Mi-2 antibodies show very strong association with dermatomyositis[9,10] with prominent features such as Gottron papules, heliotrope rash, the V sign, and shawl sign, whereas the most frequent myositis-specific autoantibodies, for example, the aminoacyl tRNA synthetases, are associated with another distinct clinical entity named antisynthetase syndrome with features including myositis, interstitial lung disease (ILD), nonerosive arthritis, Raynaud phenomenon, and skin rash on the hands, the so-called mechanic's hands.[11] To date, 8 different antisynthetase autoantibodies have been identified, of which anti-histidyl-tRNA synthetase (anti-Jo-1) autoantibodies are the most frequent, being present in 20% to 30% of patients with polymyositis or dermatomyositis. The others are anti-PL-7 directed against threonyl-tRNA synthetase, anti-PL12 directed against alanyl-tRNA synthetase, anti-KS directed against aspariginyl-tRNA synthetase, anti-OJ directed against isoleucyl-tRNA synthetase, anti-EJ directed against glycyl-tRNA synthetase, anti-Ha directed against tyrosyl-tRNA synthetase, and anti-ZO directed against anti-phenylalanyl-tRNA synthetase.[12] The most common shared clinical feature of these autoantibodies is ILD, which may precede myositis or be present even without myositis. A more recently detected autoantibody, anti-P155/140, is strongly associated with dermatomyositis and cancer as well as with juvenile dermatomyositis.[13–15] Taken together, the strong associations with distinct clinical phenotypes indicate that some of these autoantibodies are excellent clinical markers and are useful in classifying these heterogeneous disorders into homogeneous subgroups that may share pathogenic mechanisms.

The role of B cells in the pathogenesis of polymyositis and dermatomyositis is supported by the presence of B cells and plasma cell infiltrates in the muscle tissue and that immunoglobulin transcripts are among the most abundant of the immune transcripts in the muscle tissue of patients with myositis.[16,17] More recently, analyses of the variable regions' gene sequences revealed clear evidence of significant somatic mutation, isotype switching, receptor revision, codon insertion/deletion, and oligoclonal expansion, suggesting that affinity maturation had occurred within the B-cell and plasma cell populations in the muscle tissue.[18] Antigens localized to the muscle might drive a B-cell antigen-specific response in myositis, and these antigens could be autoantigens or exogenous cross-reactive antigens derived from viruses or other infectious agents. The contribution of myositis-specific autoantibodies to the disease pathogenesis is still unclear because these antibodies are often directed to ubiquitous intracellular proteins that are not muscle specific. Although the myositis-specific autoantibodies are directed against ubiquitous intracellular proteins, there is a differential organ expression of these antigens whereby histidyl-tRNA synthetase has a higher expression in the epithelial cells of the bronchi than in other healthy organs. Moreover, a proteolytically sensitive conformation of the histidyl-tRNA synthetase has been demonstrated in the lung, which might suggest that autoimmunity to histidyl-tRNA synthetase is initiated and propagated in the lung.[19] Furthermore, mice immunized with murine Jo-1 develop a striking combination of muscle and lung inflammation that replicates features of the human antisynthetase syndrome.[20] Moreover, both histidyl-tRNA synthetase and the MI-2 antigens are clearly upregulated in muscle fibers undergoing regeneration in patients with myositis, suggesting that muscle fibers may become potential targets of the immune system after trauma.[21,22] However, it is unlikely that these antibodies bind to their intracellular targets and contribute to significant tissue damage in myositis, but they could be involved in the disease pathogenesis in other ways by modulating the muscle microenvironment.

The histidyl-tRNA synthetase autoantibodies are the most studied for potential pathogenic relevance. Presence of anti-Jo-1 antibodies is strongly associated with HLA-DRB1*0301 genotype, and a few case reports suggest that these autoantibodies precede the onset of clinical myositis or ILD[23] and that they vary in serum levels with disease activity.[24] The antibody response to histidyl-tRNA synthetase undergoes class switching, spectrotype broadening, and affinity maturation, all of which are indicators of a T-cell–dependent antigen-driven process.[25] Sera from patients with anti-Jo-1 antibodies have a type I interferon–inducing capacity, similar to anti-U1RNP and anti-SSA in systemic lupus erythematosus (SLE) and Sjögren syndrome and could thereby have a role in the pathogenesis by activating the type I interferon system, which could have several roles in autoimmune diseases as discussed later.[26] In addition, sera from patients with anti-Jo-1 antibodies induced higher expression of intercellular adhesion molecule (ICAM)-1 on microvascular endothelial cells of lungs compared with other sera from patients with myositis.[27] Thus, there is a possibility that these autoantibodies or yet unknown serum-associated factors might activate endothelial cells of microvessels and thereby facilitate homing of inflammatory cells into tissues. Presence of anti-Jo-1 antibodies is also associated with high serum levels of B-cell–activating factor, similar to what has been reported for anti-SSA in patients with SLE or Sjögren syndrome.[28] Taken together, accumulating data to date might indicate an indirect pathogenic role of anti-Jo-1 autoantibodies.

Cell-Mediated Immune Response

There are mainly 2 different patterns of distribution, location, and type of lymphocyte subsets in the muscle tissue, suggesting 2 different pathways; one is dominated by CD4$^+$ T lymphocytes, macrophages, B lymphocytes, plasma cells, and dendritic cells predominantly in perivascular and perimysial areas of tissue, which is mainly but not exclusively found in patients with dermatomyositis.[1,16] The other is dominated by CD8$^+$ T and CD4$^+$ T lymphocytes, macrophages, and dendritic cells predominantly in an endomysial distribution, with inflammatory cells sometimes invading nonnecrotic muscle fibers.[1,29,30] The latter is mainly found in patients with myositis without skin rash and polymyositis. The differences in location and inflammatory cell types suggest 2 different pathogenic pathways: one directed against blood vessels and the other directed against muscle fibers. However, these patterns are not mutually exclusive, because in some patients, these 2 patterns of inflammatory cell distribution are seen in the same specimen. The vascular involvement is in patients with dermatomyositis clearly manifested in the skin and can be clinically seen in the form of capillary nailfold changes. The capillary changes and damage are attributed to complement deposition. Capillaries in both polymyositis and dermatomyositis are often fewer per muscle area compared with those in healthy individuals, and they are often abnormally thickened and may show hyperplasia and necrosis. Likely, these morphologic changes could contribute to an ischemia that, in turn, could cause muscle fiber damage.[31–33]

The endomysial inflammatory infiltrates contain a high percentage of activated CD8[+] T lymphocytes, macrophages, and CD4[+] T lymphocytes. CD8[+] cytotoxic T lymphocytes recognize major histocompatibility complex (MHC) class I on muscle fibers and may mediate muscle fiber damage. This fact is partially supported by the evidence that (1) perforin-expressing cytotoxic T cells are seen to be oriented toward the target muscle fiber and by (2) clonal proliferation of CD8 T cells, both within the muscle, and that (3) T cell lines from patients show cytotoxicity against autologous myotubes.[34,35] In some patients, T cells are present in muscle tissue even after treatment with high doses of glucocorticoids in combination with other immunosuppressive drugs. In this context, a subset of T lymphocytes, CD28[null] T cells, are of interest. CD28[null] T cells are apoptosis-resistant T lymphocytes that are terminally differentiated and lack CD28. They are often clonally expanded and have acquired new effect or functions and upregulated a set of activating receptors mostly associated with natural killer (NK) cells. Further characterization of the T lymphocytes in polymyositis and dermatomyositis has revealed that a large proportion of CD4[+] and CD8[+] T lymphocytes both in peripheral blood and in muscle tissue are of CD28[null] T-cell phenotype.[36] They were easily stimulated to produce proinflammatory cytokines, for example, interferon-γ and tumor necrosis factor (TNF). They contain perforin and granzyme, and therefore, both CD4[+] and CD8[+] CD28[null] T cells have cytotoxic potentials, but whether they have a myocytotoxic capacity is still unknown. In polymyositis, there was an association between CD28[null] T cells and disease activity, further supporting a role of these cells in disease mechanisms. The causative factor of CD4[+] and CD8[+] CD28[null] T cells in myositis is not known. High frequencies of CD4[+] CD28[null] T cells have been found in peripheral blood in other autoimmune diseases, for example, rheumatoid arthritis, and in cardiovascular disease, whereas CD8[+] CD28[null] T cells are associated with repeated antigen stimulation and are increased in peripheral blood of individuals with chronic viral infections, such as Epstein-Barr virus, human cytomegalovirus (HCMV), and human immunodeficiency virus.[37,38] In polymyositis and dermatomyositis, both CD4[+] and CD8[+] CD28[null] T cells were strongly associated with immunity to HCMV, but a causal relationship with HCMV has not been confirmed.[36] Moreover, the specificity of the CD28[null] T cells in polymyositis and dermatomyositis is not known but should be subject of future studies.

INNATE AND NONIMMUNE MECHANISMS
Cytokines

Effector molecules (cytokines and chemokines) that are produced by muscle fibers, inflammatory cells, and endothelial cells are thought to contribute to the pathogenesis of myositis.[2] Proinflammatory cytokines such as interleukin (IL)-1α, IL-1β, TNF-α, type I interferons (interferon-α and -β), the DNA-binding nonhistone protein, high-mobility group box 1 (HMGB1), and chemokines such as the alpha-chemokines CXCL9 and CXCL10 and the beta-chemokines CCL2, CCL3, CCL4, CCL19, and CCL21 are present in the muscle tissue of patients with polymyositis and dermatomyositis.[39] Other more recently reported cytokines that may also have a role in the pathogenesis of myositis are IL-15 and IL-18, although their role needs to be further explored.[40,41] These molecules may not only amplify the immune response within the muscle microenvironment but also have a direct effect on muscle fiber function.[42,43] The relative importance of the various cytokines and chemokines in patients with myositis is still uncertain, but these molecules offer possible targets for therapy in these conditions.

One way forward to achieve increased understanding of the molecular pathways in myositis is to investigate the target organ, muscle, for molecular expression in different phases of disease and in longitudinal studies using different therapies and to relate the effects on molecular expression to the effects on clinical performance.

Interleukin-1

The most consistently found cytokines in various phases of disease, at diagnosis before and after treatment, in patients with persisting muscle weakness are IL-1α and HMGB1, both molecules that may be present not only in inflammatory cells but also in endothelial cells and muscle fibers even in the absence of inflammatory cell infiltrates. A possible direct effect of IL-1 on muscle fibers is supported by the presence of IL-1RI and IL-1RII in the muscle fiber membrane. Direct functional studies have not been published to demonstrate this effect,[44] but treatment with IL-1 receptor antagonist, anakinra, has demonstrated efficacy in occasional patients, supporting a role of IL-1 in some patients with myositis.[45] In the C-protein–induced myositis model, muscle inflammation depended on IL-1 but not on TNF, lending a further support for a role of IL-1 in myositis.[46]

Enzymes in the prostaglandin pathway have been recorded in the muscle tissue: microsomal prostaglandin E synthase 1 (mPGES-1), cyclooxygenase (COX)-1, and COX-2. Conventional immunosuppressive treatment led to a significant downregulation of COX-2 in the muscle tissue of patients with myositis, but the expression of mPGES-1 and COX-1 remained unchanged, indicating a role of these enzymes in the chronicity of polymyositis and dermatomyositis.[47] Their role in the pathogenesis of myositis is not known. IL-1β, which is markedly expressed in the muscle tissue of patients with myositis, may stimulate prostaglandin E_2 (PGE$_2$) production in skeletal muscles; therefore, PGE$_2$ expression may be a downstream effect of IL-1.

Type I Interferon System

The type I interferon system has gained much focus as having a role in propagating autoimmune diseases by its ability to break tolerance, primarily based on the clinical observation that treatment with type I interferon could induce autoimmune disease such as SLE.[48] There are also a few case reports of myositis onset during interferon treatment.[49,50] In polymyositis and dermatomyositis, a type I interferon gene signature has been observed in the muscle tissue and peripheral blood,[6,51] and the interferon gene signature in peripheral blood was associated with disease activity.[52,53] Moreover, an interferon-inducing capacity was strongly associated with anti-Jo-1 and/or anti-SSA autoantibodies, as mentioned earlier, and correlated with MHC class I expression in muscle fibers.[26] In addition, the major producer of type I interferon, plasmacytoid dendritic cells, and the interferon-inducible protein, MXA, were present in the muscle tissue of preferentially not only patients with anti-Jo-1 and anti-SSA autoantibodies but also patients with dermatomyositis without detectable antibodies, indicating 2 different mechanisms that might be linked via the interferon pathway.[6,26] Targeting type I interferon, which is now possible, seems to be an attractive treatment, at least in subgroups of patients with myositis with anti-Jo-1 or anti-SSA antibodies and some patients with dermatomyositis without these autoantibodies.

HMGB1 Protein

The alarmin HMGB1 is a ubiquitous nonhistone molecule present in all nucleated cells in which it is bound to DNA. It can be actively released from monocytes and macrophages and can be released from other cells undergoing necrosis. Extranuclear HMGB1 may have proinflammatory properties and may also have a function in muscle cell regeneration. Extracellular HMGB1 was detected in the muscle tissue of patients with polymyositis and dermatomyositis and was present even after treatment with high doses of glucocorticoids in which it was localized to the cytoplasm of muscle fibers and endothelial cells even in the absence of inflammatory infiltrates.[54] A similar expression and co-localization of HMGB1- and MHC class I–positive muscle fibers were also evident in early cases without detectable inflammatory infiltrates.[43] In these tissues, HMGB1-expressing fibers outnumbered fibers expressing MHC class I. Functional studies demonstrated that HMGB1 can induce a reversible upregulation of MHC class I in the muscle fibers. Moreover, HMGB1 exposure may cause an irreversible decrease in Ca^{2+} release from the sarcoplasmic reticulum during fatigue induced by repeated tetanic contractions, which is a proxy for muscle performance, suggesting that HMGB1 has a direct negative effect on muscle fiber contractility. Furthermore, exposure to interferon-γ induced translocation of HMGB1 to the muscle fiber sarcoplasm.[43] Therefore, HMGB1 may also be a possible endogenous molecule in muscle fibers that under inflammatory stress might be translocated from the fiber nuclei to the sarcoplasm and possibly affect MHC class I expression in muscle fibers. Hypoxia is another factor that can upregulate expression of HMGB; thus, HMGB1 could be an early inducer of skeletal muscle dysfunction in polymyositis and dermatomyositis independent of the presence of inflammatory cell infiltrates.

Hypoxia

Microvessel involvement (eg, expression of adhesion molecules and IL-1α) and loss are present in both dermatomyositis and polymyositis. Clinical symptoms and muscle fatigue commonly seen in these patients could be because of muscle tissue hypoxia.[2] A local tissue hypoxia is further supported by upregulation of vascular endothelial growth factor seen in muscle tissue and in sera of patients with polymyositis and dermatomyositis.[32] The hypoxia hypothesis is supported by the evidence that clinical improvement is observed after exercise, and magnetic resonance spectroscopic analysis showing reduced levels of energy substrates (eg, ATP and phosphocreatine) before and after a workload indicates that an acquired metabolic disturbance occurs in inflammatory myopathies, and this metabolic disturbance likely contributes to impaired performance of skeletal muscle in these patients.[55]

MHC Class I Expression in Muscle Fibers

MHC class I molecules are known to play a critical role in initiating and perpetuating antigen-specific immune responses by presenting antigenic peptides to CD8[+] T lymphocytes and by regulating the activities of NK cells. Recently, it is becoming increasingly clear that MHC class I molecules have broader nonimmune functions that are not associated with antigen presentation to lymphocytes; for example, MHC class I molecules are (1) important for the retraction of synaptic connections that normally occur during development,[56] (2) crucial for maintenance of synapses during the synaptic removal process in neurons after lesion, and the absence of MHC class I expression may impede the ability of neurons to regenerate axons,[57] and (3) important for receptor-mediated transmembrane signal transduction and cell-cell communications in multiple cell types.[58]

In normal differentiated skeletal muscle cells, MHC class I is either absent or expressed at low levels; however, they can be promptly induced by proinflammatory cytokines, for example, interferon-γ or TNF-α.[59–62] In contrast, skeletal muscle of patients with myositis shows increased expression of MHC class I not only in regenerating muscle fibers but also in nonnecrotic muscle cells.[60,63,64] The biologic significance of these observations has been explored by generating a conditional transgenic mouse model overexpressing syngenic mouse MHC class I in the skeletal muscle. These mice show many features (eg, clinical, histologic, and immunologic) that resemble those of human myositis and provide a close model of the disease in humans.[65] A series of observations in patients with human myositis and in the mouse model of myositis suggest that MHC class I molecules themselves may potentially mediate muscle fiber damage and dysfunction through innate and nonimmune mechanisms in the absence of lymphocytes: (1) MHC class I staining of muscle specimens from patients with myositis shows both a cell surface and an internal reticular pattern of reactivity, indicating that some of the MHC class I molecules may be retained in the endoplasmic reticulum (ER) of muscle fibers.[8,64,66] (2) MHC class I overexpression persists in muscle fibers in the absence of an inflammatory infiltrate.[67] (3) In vivo gene transfer of MHC class I expression plasmids attenuates muscle regeneration and differentiation,[68] and the induction of MHC class I in the skeletal muscle of the transgenic mouse model of myositis results in muscle atrophy and an intrinsic decrease in force-generating capacity.[69]

Collectively, these observations indicate that the muscle impairment and fiber damage seen in myositis may be mediated not only exclusively by CD8[+] cytotoxic T lymphocyte attack but also through nonimmunologic mechanisms such as the ER stress response and hypoxia.

ER Stress

In patients with myositis, increased expression of MHC class I in myofibers initiates a series of cell autonomous changes that lead to myofiber damage. The authors and other researchers have shown that overexpression of MHC class I on muscle fibers of patients with myositis and the transgenic mouse model of myositis results in activation of the nuclear factor (NF)-κB and ER stress response pathways.[8,70,71] The authors and other researchers have shown that NF-κB is activated and several downstream NF-κB target genes (eg, MHC class I, ICAM, and monocyte chemoattractant protein-1) are increased in human myositis specimens and in the mouse model,[8,66,71–75] suggesting that this pathway may be directly involved in muscle fiber impairment and damage in myositis. Thus, MHC class I expression in the skeletal muscle links the classic immune (through CD8 T cells) and nonimmune (ER stress) mediated mechanisms of muscle impairment and damage.[8,76] Furthermore, the role of ER stress in skeletal muscle function is explored recently using hexose-6-phosphate dehydrogenase (H6PD)–deficient mice. H6PD is an enzyme that generates nicotinamide adenine dinucleotide phosphate via the pentose phosphate pathway inside the ER, and H6PD-deficient mice have severe skeletal myopathy and exhibit fasting hypoglycemia, increased insulin sensitivity, and basal and insulin-stimulated glucose uptake in fast skeletal muscle fibers, indicating mild insensitivity to glucocorticoids. These studies also showed large intrafibrillar membranous vacuoles and abnormal triads in the affected muscle, indicating an altered redox state of sarcoplasmic reticulum that, in turn, leads to activation of unfolded protein response and myopathy.[77]

Cell Death

Although classic apoptosis is not always detected in muscle specimens, signs of muscle fiber degeneration and necrosis are characteristic histopathologic features of polymyositis and dermatomyositis that may contribute to loss of muscle performance. Some, but not all, patients develop clinical muscle atrophy, which naturally may affect muscle strength and endurance. The mechanisms that cause muscle fiber degeneration or muscle atrophy have not been clarified, and both cytotoxic cell death and an effect of disuse or a negative effect of glucocorticoids have been suggested. An increasing knowledge of the mechanisms that cause muscle cell death is important to develop targeted therapies in myositis.

Some studies showed that classic apoptotic changes are absent in skeletal muscle fibers of patients with myositis because of the expression of antiapoptotic molecules (eg, FLICE inhibitory protein and inhibitor of apoptosis) in the skeletal muscle of these patients,[78,79] indicating that other forms of cell death (eg, autophagy) may be responsible for muscle cell death in myositis. Recent literature supports that ER stress response and autophagy are interconnected, for example, endogenous ER degradation–enhancing α mannosidase-like protein 1 in nonstressed cells reaches the cytosol and is degraded by basal autophagy.[80] Although caspase-3 activation is not clearly related to myositis, it has been well demonstrated that caspase-12 is activated in the murine transgenic mouse model of myositis,[8] but its role in human skeletal muscle is still unclear. Moreover, accumulation of cell surface proteins such as MHC class I in the muscle fibers of patients with myositis may also lead to both ER stress and autophagy.[76]

The role of autophagy in myositis is unexplored. One study recently compared clinical and histologic features of muscle specimen from patients with polymyositis with those of mitochondrial disease, steroid-responsive polymyositis, and inclusion body myositis. It was observed that selective weakness in the quadriceps or finger flexors was common in PM-Mito and IBM and progressed slower in PM-Mito than in IBM and that autophagy markers LC3 and α-B-crystallin were found in PM-Mito and IBM but not in polymyositis specimens.[81] Recent studies suggest that autophagy signaling (Beclin 1 and LC3-II) is upregulated in response to denervation and may preferentially target mitochondria for degradation in the skeletal muscle and consequently loss of skeletal muscle mass.[82] Deficiency of a component of V-ATPase proton pump complex (VMA21) leads to mammalian target of rapamycin (mTOR)-dependent autophagy, vacuolation, and atrophy of skeletal muscle in cell X-linked myopathy with excessive autophagy (XMEA).[83] These findings provide clues to the perifascicular atrophic phenotype seen in muscle specimens from patients with dermatomyositis.

SUMMARY

The studies described earlier clearly indicate that the pathophysiology of myositis is complex and that multiple interconnected immune (eg, antibody and T cells) and nonimmune (eg, hypoxia, ER stress, and autophagy) mechanisms are active in the muscle microenvironment. The relative contribution of these mechanisms to muscle weakness and damage is currently unknown and may vary between patients and in different phases of the disease. Therefore, future investigations are needed to address this issue. Targeting these multiple mechanisms using combination of drugs is likely to be effective in myositis and seems to be a possibility in the future.

REFERENCES

1. Dalakas MC, Hohlfeld R. Polymyositis and dermatomyositis. Lancet 2003;362: 971–82.
2. Lundberg IE. New possibilities to achieve increased understanding of disease mechanisms in idiopathic inflammatory myopathies. Curr Opin Rheumatol 2002;14:639–42.
3. Lundberg IE. The physiology of inflammatory myopathies: an overview. Acta Physiol Scand 2001;171:207–13.

4. Nagaraju K. Immunological capabilities of skeletal muscle cells. Acta Physiol Scand 2001;171:215–23.
5. Nagaraju K. Update on immunopathogenesis in inflammatory myopathies. Curr Opin Rheumatol 2001;13:461–8.
6. Greenberg SA, Pinkus JL, Pinkus GS, et al. Interferon-alpha/beta-mediated innate immune mechanisms in dermatomyositis. Ann Neurol 2005;57:664–78.
7. Lundberg IE, Grundtman C. Developments in the scientific and clinical understanding of inflammatory myopathies. Arthritis Res Ther 2008;10:220.
8. Nagaraju K, Casciola-Rosen L, Lundberg I, et al. Activation of the endoplasmic reticulum stress response in autoimmune myositis: potential role in muscle fiber damage and dysfunction. Arthritis Rheum 2005;52:1824–35.
9. Mierau R, Dick T, Bartz-Bazzanella P, et al. Strong association of dermatomyositis-specific Mi-2 autoantibodies with a tryptophan at position 9 of the HLA-DR beta chain. Arthritis Rheum 1996;39:868–76.
10. Targoff IN, Reichlin M. The association between Mi-2 antibodies and dermatomyositis. Arthritis Rheum 1985;28:796–803.
11. Love LA, Leff RL, Fraser DD, et al. A new approach to the classification of idiopathic inflammatory myopathy: myositis-specific autoantibodies define useful homogeneous patient groups. Medicine (Baltimore) 1991;70:360–74.
12. Gunawardena H, Betteridge ZE, McHugh NJ. Myositis-specific autoantibodies: their clinical and pathogenic significance in disease expression. Rheumatology (Oxford) 2009;48:607–12.
13. Chinoy H, Fertig N, Oddis CV, et al. The diagnostic utility of myositis autoantibody testing for predicting the risk of cancer-associated myositis. Ann Rheum Dis 2007;66:1345–9.
14. Gunawardena H, Wedderburn LR, North J, et al. Clinical associations of autoantibodies to a p155/140 kDa doublet protein in juvenile dermatomyositis. Rheumatology (Oxford) 2008;47:324–8.
15. Targoff IN, Mamyrova G, Trieu EP, et al. A novel autoantibody to a 155-kd protein is associated with dermatomyositis. Arthritis Rheum 2006;54:3682–9.
16. Greenberg SA, Bradshaw EM, Pinkus JL, et al. Plasma cells in muscle in inclusion body myositis and polymyositis. Neurology 2005;65:1782–7.
17. Arahata K, Engel AG. Monoclonal antibody analysis of mononuclear cells in myopathies. I: quantitation of subsets according to diagnosis and sites of accumulation and demonstration and counts of muscle fibers invaded by T cells. Ann Neurol 1984;16(2):193–208.
18. Bradshaw EM, Orihuela A, McArdel SL, et al. A local antigen-driven humoral response is present in the inflammatory myopathies. J Immunol 2007;178:547–56.
19. Levine SM, Raben N, Xie D, et al. Novel conformation of histidyl-transfer RNA synthetase in the lung: the target tissue in Jo-1 autoantibody-associated myositis. Arthritis Rheum 2007;56:2729–39.
20. Katsumata Y, Ridgway WM, Oriss T, et al. Species-specific immune responses generated by histidyl-tRNA synthetase immunization are associated with muscle and lung inflammation. J Autoimmun 2007;29:174–86.
21. Mammen AL, Casciola-Rosen LA, Hall JC, et al. Expression of the dermatomyositis autoantigen Mi-2 in regenerating muscle. Arthritis Rheum 2009;60:3784–93.
22. Casciola-Rosen L, Nagaraju K, Plotz P, et al. Enhanced autoantigen expression in regenerating muscle cells in idiopathic inflammatory myopathy. J Exp Med 2005;201:591–601.

23. Miller FW, Waite KA, Biswas T, et al. The role of an autoantigen, histidyl-tRNA synthetase, in the induction and maintenance of autoimmunity. Proc Natl Acad Sci U S A 1990;87:9933–7.

24. Stone KB, Oddis CV, Fertig N, et al. Anti-Jo-1 antibody levels correlate with disease activity in idiopathic inflammatory myopathy. Arthritis Rheum 2007;56: 3125–31.

25. Miller FW, Twitty SA, Biswas T, et al. Origin and regulation of a disease-specific autoantibody response. Antigenic epitopes, spectrotype stability, and isotype restriction of anti-Jo-1 autoantibodies. J Clin Invest 1990;85:468–75.

26. Eloranta ML, Barbasso Helmers S, Ulfgren AK, et al. A possible mechanism for endogenous activation of the type I interferon system in myositis patients with anti-Jo-1 or anti-Ro 52/anti-Ro 60 autoantibodies. Arthritis Rheum 2007;56: 3112–24.

27. Barbasso Helmers S, Englund P, Engstrom M, et al. Sera from anti-Jo-1-positive patients with polymyositis and interstitial lung disease induce expression of inter-cellular adhesion molecule 1 in human lung endothelial cells. Arthritis Rheum 2009;60:2524–30.

28. Krystufkova O, Vallerskog T, Helmers SB, et al. Increased serum levels of B cell activating factor (BAFF) in subsets of patients with idiopathic inflammatory myop-athies. Ann Rheum Dis 2009;68:836–43.

29. Page G, Chevrel G, Miossec P. Anatomic localization of immature and mature dendritic cell subsets in dermatomyositis and polymyositis: interaction with che-mokines and Th1 cytokine-producing cells. Arthritis Rheum 2004;50:199–208.

30. Greenberg SA, Pinkus GS, Amato AA, et al. Myeloid dendritic cells in inclusion-body myositis and polymyositis. Muscle Nerve 2007;35:17–23.

31. Emslie-Smith AM, Engel AG. Microvascular changes in early and advanced der-matomyositis: a quantitative study. Ann Neurol 1990;27:343–56.

32. Grundtman C, Tham E, Ulfgren AK, et al. Vascular endothelial growth factor is highly expressed in muscle tissue of patients with polymyositis and patients with dermatomyositis. Arthritis Rheum 2008;58:3224–38.

33. Kissel JT, Mendell JR, Rammohan KW. Microvascular deposition of comple-ment membrane attack complex in dermatomyositis. N Engl J Med 1986; 314:329–34.

34. Goebels N, Michaelis D, Engelhardt M, et al. Differential expression of perforin in muscle-infiltrating T cells in polymyositis and dermatomyositis. J Clin Invest 1996; 97:2905–10.

35. Hohlfeld R, Engel AG. Coculture with autologous myotubes of cytotoxic T cells isolated from muscle in inflammatory myopathies. Ann Neurol 1991;29:498–507.

36. Fasth AE, Dastmalchi M, Rahbar A, et al. T cell infiltrates in the muscles of patients with dermatomyositis and polymyositis are dominated by CD28null T cells. J Immunol 2009;183:4792–9.

37. Warrington KJ, Kent PD, Frye RL, et al. Rheumatoid arthritis is an independent risk factor for multi-vessel coronary artery disease: a case control study. Arthritis Res Ther 2005;7:R984–91.

38. Appay V, Dunbar PR, Callan M, et al. Memory CD8+ T cells vary in differentiation phenotype in different persistent virus infections. Nat Med 2002;8(4):379–85.

39. De Paepe B, Creus KK, De Bleecker JL. Role of cytokines and chemokines in idiopathic inflammatory myopathies. Curr Opin Rheumatol 2009;21:610–6.

40. Tucci M, Quatraro C, Dammacco F, et al. Interleukin-18 overexpression as a hall-mark of the activity of autoimmune inflammatory myopathies. Clin Exp Immunol 2006;146:21–31.

41. Sugiura T, Harigai M, Kawaguchi Y, et al. Increased IL-15 production of muscle cells in polymyositis and dermatomyositis. Int Immunol 2002;14:917–24.
42. Reid MB, Lannergren J, Westerblad H. Respiratory and limb muscle weakness induced by tumor necrosis factor-alpha: involvement of muscle myofilaments. Am J Respir Crit Care Med 2002;166:479–84.
43. Grundtman C, Bruton J, Yamada T, et al. Effects of HMGB1 on in vitro responses of isolated muscle fibers and functional aspects in skeletal muscles of idiopathic inflammatory myopathies. FASEB J 2010;24:570–8.
44. Grundtman C, Salomonsson S, Dorph C, et al. Immunolocalization of interleukin-1 receptors in the sarcolemma and nuclei of skeletal muscle in patients with idiopathic inflammatory myopathies. Arthritis Rheum 2007;56:674–87.
45. Furlan A, Botsios C, Ruffatti A, et al. Antisynthetase syndrome with refractory polyarthritis and fever successfully treated with the IL-1 receptor antagonist, anakinra: a case report. Joint Bone Spine 2008;75:366–7.
46. Sugihara T, Sekine C, Nakae T, et al. A new murine model to define the critical pathologic and therapeutic mediators of polymyositis. Arthritis Rheum 2007;56: 1304–14.
47. Korotkova M, Helmers SB, Loell I, et al. Effects of immunosuppressive treatment on microsomal prostaglandin E synthase 1 and cyclooxygenases expression in muscle tissue of patients with polymyositis or dermatomyositis. Ann Rheum Dis 2008;67:1596–602.
48. Ronnblom LE, Alm GV, Oberg KE. Possible induction of systemic lupus erythematosus by interferon-alpha treatment in a patient with a malignant carcinoid tumour. J Intern Med 1990;227:207–10.
49. Kalkner KM, Ronnblom L, Karlsson Parra AK, et al. Antibodies against double-stranded DNA and development of polymyositis during treatment with interferon. QJM 1998;91:393–9.
50. Dietrich LL, Bridges AJ, Albertini MR. Dermatomyositis after interferon alpha treatment. Med Oncol 2000;17:64–9.
51. Tezak Z, Hoffman EP, Lutz JL, et al. Gene expression profiling in DQA1*0501+ children with untreated dermatomyositis: a novel model of pathogenesis. J Immunol 2002;168:4154–63.
52. Baechler EC, Bauer JW, Slattery CA, et al. An interferon signature in the peripheral blood of dermatomyositis patients is associated with disease activity. Mol Med 2007;13:59–68.
53. Walsh RJ, Kong SW, Yao Y, et al. Type I interferon-inducible gene expression in blood is present and reflects disease activity in dermatomyositis and polymyositis. Arthritis Rheum 2007;56:3784–92.
54. Ulfgren AK, Grundtman C, Borg K, et al. Down-regulation of the aberrant expression of the inflammation mediator high mobility group box chromosomal protein 1 in muscle tissue of patients with polymyositis and dermatomyositis treated with corticosteroids. Arthritis Rheum 2004;50:1586–94.
55. Park JH, Olsen NJ, King L Jr, et al. Use of magnetic resonance imaging and P-31 magnetic resonance spectroscopy to detect and quantify muscle dysfunction in the amyopathic and myopathic variants of dermatomyositis. Arthritis Rheum 1995;38:68–77.
56. Huh GS, Boulanger LM, Du H, et al. Functional requirement for class I MHC in CNS development and plasticity. Science 2000;290:2155–9.
57. Oliveira AL, Thams S, Lidman O, et al. A role for MHC class I molecules in synaptic plasticity and regeneration of neurons after axotomy. Proc Natl Acad Sci U S A 2004;101:17843–8.

58. Fishman D, Elhyany S, Segal S. Non-immune functions of MHC class I glycoproteins in normal and malignant cells. Folia Biol (Praha) 2004;50:35–42.

59. Engel AG, Arahata K, Emslie-Smith A. Immune effector mechanisms in inflammatory myopathies. Res Publ Assoc Res Nerv Ment Dis 1990;68:141–57.

60. Emslie-Smith AM, Arahata K, Engel AG. Major histocompatibility complex class I antigen expression, immunolocalization of interferon subtypes, and T cell-mediated cytotoxicity in myopathies. Hum Pathol 1989;20:224–31.

61. Hohlfeld R, Engel AG. HLA expression in myoblasts. Neurology 1991;41:2015.

62. Nagaraju K, Raben N, Merritt G, et al. A variety of cytokines and immunologically relevant surface molecules are expressed by normal human skeletal muscle cells under proinflammatory stimuli. Clin Exp Immunol 1998;113:407–14.

63. Karpati G, Pouliot Y, Carpenter S. Expression of immunoreactive major histocompatibility complex products in human skeletal muscles. Ann Neurol 1988;23:64–72.

64. Englund P, Nennesmo I, Klareskog L, et al. Interleukin-1alpha expression in capillaries and major histocompatibility complex class I expression in type II muscle fibers from polymyositis and dermatomyositis patients: important pathogenic features independent of inflammatory cell clusters in muscle tissue. Arthritis Rheum 2002;46:1044–55.

65. Nagaraju K, Raben N, Loeffler L, et al. Conditional up-regulation of MHC class I in skeletal muscle leads to self-sustaining autoimmune myositis and myositis-specific autoantibodies. Proc Natl Acad Sci U S A 2000;97:9209–14.

66. Bartoccioni E, Gallucci S, Scuderi F, et al. MHC class I, MHC class II and intercellular adhesion molecule-1 (ICAM-1) expression in inflammatory myopathies. Clin Exp Immunol 1994;95:166–72.

67. Nyberg P, Wikman AL, Nennesmo I, et al. Increased expression of interleukin 1alpha and MHC class I in muscle tissue of patients with chronic, inactive polymyositis and dermatomyositis. J Rheumatol 2000;27:940–8.

68. Pavlath GK. Regulation of class I MHC expression in skeletal muscle: deleterious effect of aberrant expression on myogenesis. J Neuroimmunol 2002;125:42–50.

69. Salomonsson S, Grundtman C, Zhang SJ, et al. Upregulation of MHC class I in transgenic mice results in reduced force-generating capacity in slow-twitch muscle. Muscle Nerve 2009;39:674–82.

70. Li CK, Knopp P, Moncrieffe H, et al. Overexpression of MHC class I heavy chain protein in young skeletal muscle leads to severe myositis. Implications for juvenile myositis. Am J Pathol 2009;175:1030–40.

71. Vattemi G, Engel WK, McFerrin J, et al. Endoplasmic reticulum stress and unfolded protein response in inclusion body myositis muscle. Am J Pathol 2004;164:1–7.

72. De Bleecker JL, Engel AG. Expression of cell adhesion molecules in inflammatory myopathies and Duchenne dystrophy. J Neuropathol Exp Neurol 1994;53:369–76.

73. Nagaraju K, Raben N, Villalba ML, et al. Costimulatory markers in muscle of patients with idiopathic inflammatory myopathies and in cultured muscle cells. Clin Immunol 1999;92:161–9.

74. Chevrel G, Granet C, Miossec P. Contribution of tumour necrosis factor alpha and interleukin (IL) 1beta to IL6 production, NF-kappaB nuclear translocation, and class I MHC expression in muscle cells: in vitro regulation with specific cytokine inhibitors. Ann Rheum Dis 2005;64:1257–62.

75. Monici MC, Aguennouz M, Mazzeo A, et al. Activation of nuclear factor-kappaB in inflammatory myopathies and Duchenne muscular dystrophy. Neurology 2003; 60:993–7.
76. Henriques-Pons A, Nagaraju K. Nonimmune mechanisms of muscle damage in myositis: role of the endoplasmic reticulum stress response and autophagy in the disease pathogenesis. Curr Opin Rheumatol 2009;21:581–7.
77. Lavery GG, Walker EA, Turan N, et al. Deletion of hexose-6-phosphate dehydrogenase activates the unfolded protein response pathway and induces skeletal myopathy. J Biol Chem 2008;283:8453–61.
78. Li M, Dalakas MC. Expression of human IAP-like protein in skeletal muscle: a possible explanation for the rare incidence of muscle fiber apoptosis in T-cell mediated inflammatory myopathies. J Neuroimmunol 2000;106:1–5.
79. Nagaraju K, Casciola-Rosen L, Rosen A, et al. The inhibition of apoptosis in myositis and in normal muscle cells. J Immunol 2000;164:5459–65.
80. Le Fourn V, Gaplovska-Kysela K, Guhl B, et al. Basal autophagy is involved in the degradation of the ERAD component EDEM1. Cell Mol Life Sci 2009;66:1434–45.
81. Temiz P, Weihl CC, Pestronk A. Inflammatory myopathies with mitochondrial pathology and protein aggregates. J Neurol Sci 2009;278:25–9.
82. O'Leary MF, Hood DA. Denervation-induced oxidative stress and autophagy signaling in muscle. Autophagy 2009;5:230–1.
83. Ramachandran N, Munteanu I, Wang P, et al. VMA21 deficiency causes an autophagic myopathy by compromising V-ATPase activity and lysosomal acidification. Cell 2009;137:235–46.

Inclusion Body Myositis: Diagnosis, Pathogenesis, and Treatment Options

Guillermo E. Solorzano, MD*, Lawrence H. Phillips II, MD

KEYWORDS

• Inclusion body myositis • Pathogenesis • Treatment

Sporadic inclusion body myositis (sIBM) is but one of the inflammatory myopathies. The inflammatory myopathies are characterized by varying degrees of muscle weakness in the setting of endomysial inflammation and elevations in creatine kinase.[1] sIBM is the most common inflammatory myopathy in people older than 50 years.[2] The term *sporadic* inclusion body myositis is used here to distinguish it from *hereditary* inclusion body *myopathy* (hIBM), which is a distinct disorder that is not associated with muscle inflammation and presents with a different distribution of weakness. hIBM is not discussed in this article. The interested reader may find it useful to read a review by Askanas and Engel.[3]

For the sake of simplicity, the remainder of this article uses the term inclusion body myositis (IBM) to mean sporadic inclusion body myositis. This review focuses on the clinical presentation of IBM, and discusses its pathogenesis and treatment options.

EPIDEMIOLOGY

Relatively few studies have looked at the epidemiology of IBM. The prevalence of IBM in the Netherlands is 4.9 cases per million inhabitants.[4] In Australia, it is reported at 9.3 cases per million inhabitants.[5] In a study population of 9 Caucasian individuals diagnosed with IBM in Olmsted County, Minnesota, researchers estimated the incidence of IBM, adjusted for sex and age to the 2000 US Census population, at 7.9 cases per million inhabitants.[6] In the same study, they estimated the prevalence to be 70 cases per million inhabitants.[6] However, the epidemiology of IBM in non-Caucasian populations is far different. In a study of Mesoamerican, self-classified mestizos, no cases of IBM were reported among the 98 adults diagnosed with an idiopathic inflammatory myopathy.[7]

The authors have nothing to disclose.
Department of Neurology, University of Virginia School of Medicine, PO Box 800394, Charlottesville, VA 22908-0394, USA
* Corresponding author.
E-mail address: ges3b@virginia.edu

Rheum Dis Clin N Am 37 (2011) 173–183
doi:10.1016/j.rdc.2011.01.003
0889-857X/11/$ – see front matter © 2011 Elsevier Inc. All rights reserved.

Differences in worldwide distribution of IBM may be related to genetic or environmental factors. Genetic susceptibility studies have found a strong association between IBM and HLA-DR3 (up to 75% of IBM cases in certain populations).[8] The 8.1 MHC ancestral haplotype (a conserved combination of alleles including HLA-A*01, -B*0801, -DRB1*0301, -DQB1*0201, -DQA1*05) is also associated with IBM in Australian, Dutch and North American white populations.[9] In Japanese individuals, IBM appears to be related to the 52.1 ancestral haplotype (which includes HLA-B*5201 and HLA-DRB*1502).[10] Therefore, although a genetic linkage is evident, more studies are necessary to better understand the role of genes in IBM.

CLINICAL FEATURES

IBM tends to primarily affect individuals older than 50 years, but it should be considered in patients with appropriate symptoms who are older than 30.[11] It is more common in men than women. The disease presents insidiously, with a reported mean time to diagnosis ranging from 1 to 9 years.[12,13] IBM characteristically presents with quadriceps and forearm flexor (especially the flexor digitorum profundus) weakness.[1,8,12–14] Quadriceps and forearm atrophy may be seen as the presenting feature.[8] A finding that helps distinguish IBM from other inflammatory myopathies, such as dermatomyositis and polymyositis, is an asymmetric distribution of weakness.[8,12,13]

Lower extremity complaints come typically in the form of difficulty arising from chairs, and walking upstairs or downstairs. As the disease progresses, lower extremity weakness leads to frequent falls.[8] Although one can conclude that falls in IBM patients occur as a result of proximal muscle weakness, distal lower extremity weakness occurs as well. In fact, foot drop is a recognized feature of IBM.[8,12,14,15]

Upper extremity weakness manifests as difficulty with fine motor skills, including buttoning buttons, zipping zippers, or opening jars, given the finger flexor weakness found in this disorder. Some clinicians note that a weak handshake (suggestive of weakness of grip) may be a clue to the diagnosis.[1]

Dysphagia, caused by esophageal and pharyngeal muscle involvement, is reported in anywhere from 40% to 60% of patients.[8,14–16] It may even be the presenting symptom.[17] Dysphagia in IBM is reported to affect nutrition in some, but not all patients.[18] Some groups have noted that dysphagia is underreported by patients.[19]

Other muscle groups may be affected in IBM. Facial weakness occurs in about one-third of cases.[15] Unusual presentations of IBM have also been reported, including involvement of only the erector spinae muscles.[20]

Peripheral neuropathy may be found on clinical neurophysiological testing.[15] In a series of 12 patients with IBM, morphometric studies of sural nerve biopsies demonstrated varying reductions in myelinated fibers indicative of a neuropathic process.[21] However, the neuropathy observed in patients with IBM is largely asymptomatic.[15] Comorbid autoimmune diseases, such as systemic lupus erythematosus, Sjögren syndrome, scleroderma, and variable immunodeficiency have been reported in IBM patients.[22]

In general, IBM is a slowly progressive disease. In a prospective study by Rose and colleagues[23] of 11 IBM patients, quantitative strength testing demonstrated a 4% decline over 6 months. However, the investigators reported that 4 of their 11 patients demonstrated no change. In a retrospective trial, the rate of functional decline of patients, measured by time to use of an assistive device, was faster in those patients diagnosed after age 60 years compared with those diagnosed when they were younger.[24]

LABORATORY FINDINGS

Elevations in creatine kinase (CK) are common, but they are generally less than 12 times the upper limit of normal.[11] Autoantibodies associated with myositis are usually not found in IBM patients.[22] Paraproteinemia is overrepresented in IBM patients when compared with age-matched controls.[25]

ELECTRODIAGNOSTIC FINDINGS

Electromyographic study of IBM patients demonstrates increased insertional activity and short-duration, polyphasic motor unit potentials (MUAPs) with early recruitment.[15,26] In one series of 30 patients with biopsy-proven IBM, about a third of the patients demonstrated a mixed pattern of what are commonly referred to as "neurogenic" and "myopathic" MUAPs.[27] Some authorities ascribe these "neurogenic" potentials to a secondary process.[15] As previously noted, nerve conduction studies in IBM patients are consistent with a superimposed peripheral neuropathy.[15]

DIAGNOSIS

IBM presents insidiously and manifests with atrophy of forearm and quadriceps muscles. These findings, along with electrodiagnostic and pathologic findings, have been used to establish diagnostic criteria. One set of criteria were put forth by Griggs and colleagues.[11] More recently, modified IBM criteria were posed during an IBM workshop by the MRC Center for Neuromuscular Diseases (**Box 1**).[28] The purpose of modifying the criteria was to help in the diagnosis of patients who clinically appear to have IBM but do not have the pathologic criteria set forth by earlier groups. One should note that both sets of proposed criteria do not include the use of radiographic studies. Magnetic resonance imaging (MRI) of muscle in IBM patients demonstrates involvement of the quadriceps femoris and the medial gastrocnemii along with forearm flexors (especially the flexor digitorum profundus).[12] Some believe that MRI is of limited diagnostic value,[1] as quantitative muscle testing revealed weakness in muscles that did not have signal changes on MRI.[12]

The most helpful diagnostic test of IBM is muscle biopsy. Which muscle to biopsy depends on the clinical presentation. A good rule of thumb is to avoid muscles that are at or are less than antigravity strength, as the biopsy will most likely show fibrosis. Because IBM tends to affect the quadriceps muscles, a muscle often biopsied is the vastus lateralis. However, if the muscle is too atrophied, other muscles including the biceps brachii, deltoid, or even the tibialis anterior can be biopsied.[15] The specific findings seen on muscle biopsy are discussed at greater length in the histopathology section of this review.

DIFFERENTIAL DIAGNOSIS

Perhaps the most common misdiagnosis of a patient with IBM is polymyositis. The error stems partially from the misinformed notion that elevations in CK accompanied by muscle weakness are characteristics only of polymyositis. As stated previously, the pattern of muscle involvement can help guide a clinician toward the right diagnostic path. It is important to mention that the characteristic findings of IBM are not always seen on muscle biopsy. In the authors' experience it is not uncommon to receive a patient's muscle pathology report with a diagnosis of "polymyositis" when clinically the patient appears to have IBM.

Given the "neurogenic" findings seen on electrodiagnostic studies along with the asymmetric distribution of weakness, amyotrophic lateral sclerosis (ALS) is in the

---

Box 1
Proposed modified IBM diagnostic criteria

Pathologically Defined IBM

    Conforming to the Griggs criteria[11]: invasion of non-necrotic fibers by mononuclear cells and rimmed vacuoles, and either intracellular amyloid deposits or 15- to 18-nm filaments.

Clinically Defined IBM

    Clinical Features

        Duration of weakness >12 months

        Age >35 years

        Weakness of finger flexion > shoulder abduction *AND* of knee extension > hip flexion

    Pathologic Features

        Invasion of non-necrotic fibers by mononuclear cells or rimmed vacuoles or increased MHC-1, but no intracellular amyloid deposits or 15- to 18-nm filaments

Possible IBM

    Clinical Criteria

        Duration of weakness >12 months

        Age >35 years

        Weakness of finger flexion > shoulder abduction *OR* of knee extension > hip flexion

    Pathologic Criteria

        Invasion of non-necrotic fibers by mononuclear cells or rimmed vacuoles or increased MHC-1, but no intracellular amyloid deposits or 15-to 18-nm filaments

From Hilton-Jones D, Miller A, Parton M, et al. Inclusion body myositis. MRC Centre for Neuromuscular Diseases, IBM workshop, London, 13 June 2008. Neuromuscul Disord 20:143; Copyright 2009, with permission from Elsevier.

---

differential for IBM. Important features of ALS that help to distinguish it from IBM are hyperreflexia, severe dysphagia, fasciculations, and cramping. Furthermore, atrophy in ALS tends to affect intrinsic muscles of the hand, the so-called split-hand syndrome,[29] rather than the deep finger flexors.

As briefly mentioned in the introduction, hIBMs are a group of inherited, usually noninflammatory myopathies that affect distal musculature and share some common pathologic characteristics with IBM (mainly vacuolar changes on muscle biopsy).[3]

Rimmed vacuoles on muscle biopsy of patients with IBM are not specific to the disease. Vacuolar changes are seen in a variety of muscle disorders including oculopharyngeal muscular dystrophy, oculopharyngodistal myopathy, distal myopathy with rimmed vacuoles, inclusion body myopathy, and myofibrillar myopathy.[30,31] More recently, rimmed vacuoles have been reported in a case series of patients with facioscapulohumeral muscular dystrophy.[32] There is at least one case report of rimmed vacuoles in a case of dermatomyositis.[33]

HISTOPATHOLOGY

A "definite" diagnosis of IBM includes finding particular abnormalities on muscle biopsy.[11] Features seen include: (1) mononuclear cell invasion of non-necrotic endomysial fibers; (2) intracellular amyloid deposits seen with Congo Red staining techniques; (3) eosinophilic intracytoplasmic inclusions; (4) rimmed vacuoles; and (5) loss of cyclooxygenase (COX) staining of certain fibers.[8]

Immunohistochemical staining of IBM muscle demonstrates that mononuclear infiltrates are composed of CD8[+] T cells.[34] MHC-1 expression in muscle fibers is also a feature of IBM muscle pathology.[8] Myeloid rather than plasmacytoid dendritic cells are reported to surround non-necrotic areas in affected muscle fibers.[35] These findings suggest a role for adaptive immunity in the pathophysiology of IBM. It is interesting that through immunohistochemical techniques, using markers for CD138, plasma cells have been reported in muscle biopsies of IBM patients.[36]

Rimmed vacuoles, round or polygonal structures that are surrounded by a basophilic rim on hematoxylin-eosin stains (**Fig. 1**), are a feature of IBM muscle. The make-up of these structures is of interest. Nuclear membrane proteins, including emerin and lamin A/C, are reported to line these structures.[37,38] Other myonuclear-associated structures such as histone-1[38] and valosin-containing protein[39] are also found in the lining of rimmed vacuoles. Immunostaining for TDP-43, a nucleic acid binding protein, is reported to yield an abnormal distribution in the cytoplasm of IBM muscle.[40] In fact, Salajegheh and colleagues[40] reported that more than 1% of myofibers stained for TDP-43 outside of the nucleus, and they were 91% sensitive and 100% specific for the diagnosis of IBM in their study of 50 patients.

Cytoplasmic inclusions are another feature of muscle affected by IBM. Inclusions are reportedly seen by stains for ubiquitin.[41] The use of an antibody directed against phosphorylated tau (SMI-31) has been reported to help visualize cytoplasmic inclusions that are not otherwise seen by light microscopy (see **Fig. 1**).[42]

At specialized centers, electron microscopy can help in the diagnosis of IBM. The cytoplasmic inclusions reported to stain with the SMI-31 antibodies are seen as 15- to 21-nm paired helical filaments or tubulofilaments.[42] Other ultrastructural findings of IBM muscle include 6- to 10-nm amyloid-like filaments.[11]

PATHOGENESIS

Despite years of dedicated research, the pathogenesis of IBM remains unknown. Immunohistochemical studies as well as ultrastructural studies have yielded postulated mechanisms for the pathogenesis of IBM. Some of the findings point toward an immune-mediated cause, whereas others may indicate a degenerative process.

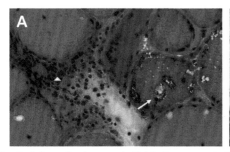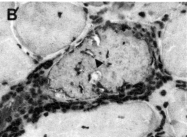

Fig. 1. Selected microscopic fields from muscle biopsy of a patient with IBM. In (*panel A*) muscle is stained with hematoxylin and eosin. The white arrow points to a rimmed vacuole. The white arrowhead is directed at the mononuclear endomysial inflammatory infiltrates. The (*panel B*) demonstrates lower field demonstrates a muscle fiber stained with SMI-31. It shows aggregates surrounding rimmed vacuoles (*black arrowhead*), as well as aggregates scattered within the muscle fiber. (*Courtesy of* Katherine Lindstrom, MD.)

The presence of CD8[+] T cells invading non-necrotic fibers has prompted some investigators to think of IBM as a primarily immune-mediated disorder.[43,44] Evidence supportive of this hypothesis includes identification of clonally expanded T cells in invaded myofibers.[45] Furthermore, electron microscopy studies demonstrate that invasion of non-necrotic muscle fibers by T cells occurs more frequently than other pathologic hallmarks of the disease, such as rimmed vacuoles and congophilic amyloid inclusions.[46] Upregulation of inducible costimulator and its ligand add credence to the role of muscle fibers acting as antigen-presenting cells in the pathogenesis of IBM.[47] This opinion is further supported by the finding of myeloid dendritic cells, which serve as antigen-presenting cells, in tissue samples of IBM affected muscle.[35] The role of plasma cells, identified in IBM affected muscle via microarray studies, is also suggestive of a possible immune-mediated mechanism.[36] Furthermore, there is evidence suggestive of a humoral antigen-driven response in tissue samples from IBM patients.[48] The importance of the overrepresentation of paraproteinemias in IBM patients is also of unclear significance.[25]

The lack of clinical response, despite reduced evidence of inflammation, to immunomodulatory therapy[49] argues against IBM as a primarily immune-mediated disease. The lack of clinical response to immunomodulatory therapies has been replicated by many groups.[49–51]

The degenerative pathogenesis model of IBM stems from the identification of protein aggregates (beta-amyloid, phosphorylated tau, presenilin, and parkin, among others) often associated with other neurodegenerative diseases.[52–54] These aggregates are postulated to occur due to protein misfolding, thus leading to accumulation of aberrant proteins.[53] Protein accumulation is thought to lead to failure of cellular processes geared toward disposing of misfolded proteins.[54] The postulated mechanisms that falter are the 26 S proteasome system, various heat shock proteins, and disturbances in autophagy.[54–56] Proponents of this theory postulate that the inflammatory changes seen are secondary to aberrant protein accumulation. Critics of the postulated degenerative theories note the lack of critically supported data that demonstrate the presence of phosphorylated tau in IBM muscle specimens.[57]

Links between the mainly immune-mediated and the mainly degenerative theories exist. Colocalization between the proinflammatory cytokine 1LB and the amyloid precursor protein in IBM muscle[58] suggests such a link. In a murine experimental model of inflammatory myopathy, researchers demonstrated evidence of inflammation leading to tau pathology.[59] However, other groups argue against such causal links.[60]

The interplay between the two major theories regarding the pathogenesis of IBM remains highly debated. The role of mitochondrial DNA mutations, which occur with greater frequency in patients with IBM when compared with age-matched controls, may be a secondary finding.[61] Myonuclear degeneration, as evidenced by the presence of myonuclear proteins in rimmed vacuoles,[37,40] and its role in the pathogenesis of inclusion body myositis is unclear. On a final note, there is a body of literature suggesting that viruses play a role, such as the human immunodeficiency virus, as possible agents in the pathogenesis of IBM.[62]

TREATMENT

There are no proven pharmacologic treatments for IBM. Given the inflammatory infiltrates seen in IBM muscle, oral steroids have been used to treat the disease. In a series of 8 patients followed from 6 to 24 months, Barohn and colleagues[49] demonstrated reduced inflammatory infiltrates and levels of CK in patients but no improvements in strength. The use of intravenous immunoglobulin (IVIg) has met with mixed results. Investigators report some improvement in dysphagia but no significant improvement in strength.[6,51,63] The combination of prednisone and IVIg also proved to be ineffective.[64] A randomized controlled trial of weekly methotrexate failed to demonstrate improvement.[50]

Given the potential involvement of T lymphocytes in IBM, an open-label, randomized pilot study using Anti–T-lymphocyte globulin (ATG) was conducted, but failed to provide clear benefit.[65] In a proof-of-principle trial, Dalakas and colleagues[66] reported that patients' strength improved 6 months after treatment with alemtuzumab (a humanized-monoclonal antibody against CD52) when compared with a pretreatment observation period. However, some concerns over the results have been raised by other investigators.[67]

A pilot trial using the anti–tumor necrosis factor-α drug etanercept showed promise by demonstrating improved handgrip strength after 12 months.[68] This study has prompted an ongoing double-blind, placebo-controlled trial of etanercept (see clinicaltrials.gov for details).

A randomized trial of high-dose beta interferon-1a (60 μg intramuscularly, weekly) demonstrated significant improvement in grip strength. However, the study failed to show statistical significance in other measured outcomes.[69]

Ongoing trials aimed at finding treatments for IBM include the aforementioned etanercept trial as well as a recently closed pilot trial studying the use of lithium (see clinicaltrials.gov). The rationale behind the use of lithium is that it serves as an inducer of autophagy, thereby improving clearance of misfolded proteins.[70] Furthermore, in a transgenic mouse model of inflammatory myopathy treated with lithium for 6 months, animals demonstrated a trend toward improved motor performance, although results were not statistically significant.[59] With the putative role of heat shock protein abnormalities playing a role in the pathogenesis of IBM, there is a trial of arimoclomol, a heat shock protein inducer, for the treatment of IBM (see clinicaltrials.gov).

SUMMARY

IBM is the most common acquired myopathy in people older than 50 years. It typically presents with knee extensor and finger flexor weakness. Asymmetric weakness is not unusual. Associated clinical findings include distal lower extremity weakness and dysphagia. The diagnosis of IBM is made with the aid of muscle pathology, but the clinical impression is very important, as widely accepted pathologic hallmarks are neither always present nor specific to the disease. The pathogenesis of IBM remains unclear. Pharmacotherapy for this condition has not proved to be efficacious.

REFERENCES

1. Dalakas MC. Sporadic inclusion body myositis—diagnosis, pathogenesis and therapeutic strategies. Nat Clin Pract Neurol 2006;2(8):437–47.
2. Needham M, Mastaglia FL. Sporadic inclusion body myositis: a continuing puzzle. Neuromuscul Disord 2008;18(1):6–16.
3. Askanas V, Engel WK. Sporadic inclusion-body myositis and hereditary inclusion-body myopathies: current concepts of diagnosis and pathogenesis. Curr Opin Rheumatol 1998;10(6):530–42.
4. Badrising UA, Maat-Schieman M, van Duinen SG, et al. Epidemiology of inclusion body myositis in the Netherlands: a nationwide study. Neurology 2000;55(9): 1385–7.

5. Phillips BA, Zilko PJ, Mastaglia FL. Prevalence of sporadic inclusion body myositis in Western Australia. Muscle Nerve 2000;23(6):970–2.

6. Wilson FC, Ytterberg SR, St Sauver JL, et al. Epidemiology of sporadic inclusion body myositis and polymyositis in Olmsted County, Minnesota. J Rheumatol 2008;35(3):445–7.

7. Shamim EA, Rider LG, Pandey JP, et al. Differences in idiopathic inflammatory myopathy phenotypes and genotypes between Mesoamerican Mestizos and North American Caucasians: ethnogeographic influences in the genetics and clinical expression of myositis. Arthritis Rheum 2002;46(7):1885–93.

8. Needham M, Mastaglia FL. Inclusion body myositis: current pathogenetic concepts and diagnostic and therapeutic approaches. Lancet Neurol 2007; 6(7):620–31.

9. Needham M, Mastaglia FL, Garlepp MJ. Genetics of inclusion-body myositis. Muscle Nerve 2007;35(5):549–61.

10. Scott AP, Allcock RJ, Mastaglia F, et al. Sporadic inclusion body myositis in Japanese is associated with the MHC ancestral haplotype 52.1. Neuromuscul Disord 2006;16(5):311–5.

11. Griggs RC, Askanas V, DiMauro S, et al. Inclusion body myositis and myopathies. Ann Neurol 1995;38(5):705–13.

12. Phillips BA, Cala LA, Thickbroom GW, et al. Patterns of muscle involvement in inclusion body myositis: clinical and magnetic resonance imaging study. Muscle Nerve 2001;24(11):1526–34.

13. Amato AA, Gronseth GS, Jackson CE, et al. Inclusion body myositis: clinical and pathological boundaries. Ann Neurol 1996;40(4):581–6.

14. Engel WK, Askanas V. Inclusion-body myositis: clinical, diagnostic, and pathologic aspects. Neurology 2006;66(2 Suppl 1):S20–9.

15. Amato AA, Barohn RJ. Inclusion body myositis: old and new concepts. J Neurol Neurosurg Psychiatry 2009;80(11):1186–93.

16. Tawil R, Griggs RC. Inclusion body myositis. Curr Opin Rheumatol 2002;14(6): 653–7.

17. Oh TH, Brumfield KA, Hoskin TL, et al. Dysphagia in inflammatory myopathy: clinical characteristics, treatment strategies, and outcome in 62 patients. Mayo Clin Proc 2007;82(4):441–7.

18. Houser SM, Calabrese LH, Strome M. Dysphagia in patients with inclusion body myositis. Laryngoscope 1998;108(7):1001–5.

19. Cox FM, Verschuuren JJ, Verbist BM, et al. Detecting dysphagia in inclusion body myositis. J Neurol 2009;256(12):2009–13.

20. Hund E, Heckl R, Goebel HH, et al. Inclusion body myositis presenting with isolated erector spinae paresis. Neurology 1995;45(5):993–4.

21. Hermanns B, Molnar M, Schroder JM. Peripheral neuropathy associated with hereditary and sporadic inclusion body myositis: confirmation by electron microscopy and morphometry. J Neurol Sci 2000;179(S1/2):92–102.

22. Koffman BM, Rugiero M, Dalakas MC. Immune-mediated conditions and antibodies associated with sporadic inclusion body myositis. Muscle Nerve 1998; 21(1):115–7.

23. Rose MR, McDermott MP, Thornton CA, et al. A prospective natural history study of inclusion body myositis: implications for clinical trials. Neurology 2001;57(3):548–50.

24. Peng A, Koffman BM, Malley JD, et al. Disease progression in sporadic inclusion body myositis: observations in 78 patients. Neurology 2000;55(2):296–8.

25. Dalakas MC, Illa I, Gallardo E, et al. Inclusion body myositis and paraproteinemia: incidence and immunopathologic correlations. Ann Neurol 1997;41(1):100–4.

26. Lotz BP, Engel AG, Nishino H, et al. Inclusion body myositis. Observations in 40 patients. Brain 1989;112(Pt 3):727–47.
27. Joy JL, Oh SJ, Baysal AI. Electrophysiological spectrum of inclusion body myositis. Muscle Nerve 1990;13(10):949–51.
28. Hilton-Jones D, Miller A, Parton M, et al. Inclusion body myositis: MRC Centre for Neuromuscular Diseases, IBM workshop, London, 13 June 2008. Neuromuscul Disord 2010;20(2):142–7.
29. Wilbourn AJ. The "split hand syndrome". Muscle Nerve 2000;23(1):138.
30. Nonaka I, Murakami N, Suzuki Y, et al. Distal myopathy with rimmed vacuoles. Neuromuscul Disord 1998;8(5):333–7.
31. Saperstein DS, Amato AA, Barohn RJ. Clinical and genetic aspects of distal myopathies. Muscle Nerve 2001;24(11):1440–50.
32. Reilich P, Schramm N, Schoser B, et al. Facioscapulohumeral muscular dystrophy presenting with unusual phenotypes and atypical morphological features of vacuolar myopathy. J Neurol 2010;257(7):1108–18.
33. Layzer R, Lee HS, Iverson D, et al. Dermatomyositis with inclusion body myositis pathology. Muscle Nerve 2009;40(3):469–71.
34. Dalakas MC. Muscle biopsy findings in inflammatory myopathies. Rheum Dis Clin North Am 2002;28(4):779–98, vi.
35. Greenberg SA, Pinkus GS, Amato AA, et al. Myeloid dendritic cells in inclusion-body myositis and polymyositis. Muscle Nerve 2007;35(1):17–23.
36. Greenberg SA, Bradshaw EM, Pinkus JL, et al. Plasma cells in muscle in inclusion body myositis and polymyositis. Neurology 2005;65(11):1782–7.
37. Greenberg SA, Pinkus JL, Amato AA. Nuclear membrane proteins are present within rimmed vacuoles in inclusion-body myositis. Muscle Nerve 2006;34(4):406–16.
38. Nakano S, Shinde A, Fujita K, et al. Histone H1 is released from myonuclei and present in rimmed vacuoles with DNA in inclusion body myositis. Neuromuscul Disord 2008;18(1):27–33.
39. Greenberg SA, Watts GD, Kimonis VE, et al. Nuclear localization of valosin-containing protein in normal muscle and muscle affected by inclusion-body myositis. Muscle Nerve 2007;36(4):447–54.
40. Salajegheh M, Pinkus JL, Taylor JP, et al. Sarcoplasmic redistribution of nuclear TDP-43 in inclusion body myositis. Muscle Nerve 2009;40(1):19–31.
41. Askanas V, Serdaroglu P, Engel WK, et al. Immunolocalization of ubiquitin in muscle biopsies of patients with inclusion body myositis and oculopharyngeal muscular dystrophy. Neurosci Lett 1991;130(1):73–6.
42. Askanas V, Alvarez RB, Mirabella M, et al. Use of anti-neurofilament antibody to identify paired-helical filaments in inclusion-body myositis. Ann Neurol 1996;39(3):389–91.
43. Arahata K, Engel AG. Monoclonal antibody analysis of mononuclear cells in myopathies. I: quantitation of subsets according to diagnosis and sites of accumulation and demonstration and counts of muscle fibers invaded by T cells. Ann Neurol 1984;16(2):193–208.
44. Engel AG, Arahata K. Monoclonal antibody analysis of mononuclear cells in myopathies. II: phenotypes of autoinvasive cells in polymyositis and inclusion body myositis. Ann Neurol 1984;16(2):209–15.
45. Salajegheh M, Rakocevic G, Raju R, et al. T cell receptor profiling in muscle and blood lymphocytes in sporadic inclusion body myositis. Neurology 2007;69(17):1672–9.
46. Pruitt JN 2nd, Showalter CJ, Engel AG. Sporadic inclusion body myositis: counts of different types of abnormal fibers. Ann Neurol 1996;39(1):139–43.

47. Schmidt J, Rakocevic G, Raju R, et al. Upregulated inducible co-stimulator (ICOS) and ICOS-ligand in inclusion body myositis muscle: significance for CD8+ T cell cytotoxicity. Brain 2004;127(Pt 5):1182–90.

48. Bradshaw EM, Orihuela A, McArdel SL, et al. A local antigen-driven humoral response is present in the inflammatory myopathies. J Immunol 2007;178(1): 547–56.

49. Barohn RJ, Amato AA, Sahenk Z, et al. Inclusion body myositis: explanation for poor response to immunosuppressive therapy. Neurology 1995;45(7):1302–4.

50. Badrising UA, Maat-Schieman ML, Ferrari MD, et al. Comparison of weakness progression in inclusion body myositis during treatment with methotrexate or placebo. Ann Neurol 2002;51(3):369–72.

51. Walter MC, Lochmuller H, Toepfer M, et al. High-dose immunoglobulin therapy in sporadic inclusion body myositis: a double-blind, placebo-controlled study. J Neurol 2000;247(1):22–8.

52. Askanas V, Engel WK. Proposed pathogenetic cascade of inclusion-body myositis: importance of amyloid-beta, misfolded proteins, predisposing genes, and aging. Curr Opin Rheumatol 2003;15(6):737–44.

53. Askanas V, Engel WK. Inclusion-body myositis: a myodegenerative conformational disorder associated with Abeta, protein misfolding, and proteasome inhibition. Neurology 2006;66(2 Suppl 1):S39–48.

54. Askanas V, Engel WK, Nogalska A. Inclusion body myositis: a degenerative muscle disease associated with intra-muscle fiber multi-protein aggregates, proteasome inhibition, endoplasmic reticulum stress and decreased lysosomal degradation. Brain Pathol 2009;19(3):493–506.

55. Muth IE, Barthel K, Bahr M, et al. Proinflammatory cell stress in sporadic inclusion body myositis muscle: overexpression of alphaB-crystallin is associated with amyloid precursor protein and accumulation of beta-amyloid. J Neurol Neurosurg Psychiatry 2009;80(12):1344–9.

56. Lunemann JD, Schmidt J, Schmid D, et al. Beta-amyloid is a substrate of autophagy in sporadic inclusion body myositis. Ann Neurol 2007;61(5):476–83.

57. Salajegheh M, Pinkus JL, Nazareno R, et al. Nature of "Tau" immunoreactivity in normal myonuclei and inclusion body myositis. Muscle Nerve 2009;40(4):520–8.

58. Schmidt J, Barthel K, Wrede A, et al. Interrelation of inflammation and APP in sIBM: IL-1 beta induces accumulation of beta-amyloid in skeletal muscle. Brain 2008;131(Pt 5):1228–40.

59. Kitazawa M, Trinh DN, LaFerla FM. Inflammation induces tau pathology in inclusion body myositis model via glycogen synthase kinase-3beta. Ann Neurol 2008; 64(1):15–24.

60. Greenberg SA. Comment on 'Interrelation of inflammation and APP in sIBM: IL-1beta induces accumulation of beta-amyloid in skeletal muscle'. Brain 2009; 132(Pt 4):e106 [author reply: e107].

61. Oldfors A, Moslemi AR, Fyhr IM, et al. Mitochondrial DNA deletions in muscle fibers in inclusion body myositis. J Neuropathol Exp Neurol 1995;54(4):581–7.

62. Dalakas MC, Rakocevic G, Shatunov A, et al. Inclusion body myositis with human immunodeficiency virus infection: four cases with clonal expansion of viral-specific T cells. Ann Neurol 2007;61(5):466–75.

63. Dalakas MC, Sonies B, Dambrosia J, et al. Treatment of inclusion-body myositis with IVIg: a double-blind, placebo-controlled study. Neurology 1997;48(3):712–6.

64. Dalakas MC, Koffman B, Fujii M, et al. A controlled study of intravenous immunoglobulin combined with prednisone in the treatment of IBM. Neurology 2001; 56(3):323–7.

65. Lindberg C, Trysberg E, Tarkowski A, et al. Anti-T-lymphocyte globulin treatment in inclusion body myositis: a randomized pilot study. Neurology 2003;61(2): 260–2.
66. Dalakas MC, Rakocevic G, Schmidt J, et al. Effect of alemtuzumab (CAMPATH 1-H) in patients with inclusion-body myositis. Brain 2009;132(Pt 6):1536–44.
67. Greenberg SA. Comment on alemtuzumab and inclusion body myositis. Brain 2010;133(Pt 5):e135.
68. Barohn RJ, Herbelin L, Kissel JT, et al. Pilot trial of etanercept in the treatment of inclusion-body myositis. Neurology 2006;66(2 Suppl 1):S123–4.
69. Muscle Study Group. Randomized pilot trial of high-dose betaINF-1a in patients with inclusion body myositis. Neurology 2004;63(4):718–20.
70. Sarkar S, Floto RA, Berger Z, et al. Lithium induces autophagy by inhibiting inositol monophosphatase. J Cell Biol 2005;170(7):1101–11.

Paraneoplastic Muscle Disease

Alan N. Baer, MD

KEYWORDS

- Malignancy • Myopathy • Dermatomyositis • Polymyositis
- Paraneoplastic • Eaton-Lambert syndrome • Myasthenia gravis
- Stiff person syndrome

Skeletal muscle disease may arise in the setting of malignancy. The potential mechanisms are varied and may include direct invasion of the muscle by an adjacent tumor, the rare occurrence of a skeletal muscle metastasis, muscle injury from chemotherapy or infection, dysfunction from metabolic derangements, and wasting as a result of tumor-related cachexia. The term paraneoplastic is applied when none of these mechanisms are applicable.[1] In paraneoplastic muscle disease, the malignancy may remotely affect neuromuscular transmission or incite muscle inflammation or necrosis. In several of these diseases, an autoimmune basis for the muscle disease has been established and has become a defining feature.[2,3] These paraneoplastic muscle diseases may be the first manifestation of a malignancy, and their diagnosis thus demands a vigilant search for an underlying tumor. This article is focused on inflammatory and necrotizing myopathies and disorders of neuromuscular transmission that may arise in the setting of malignancy and are considered paraneoplastic phenomena.

DERMATOMYOSITIS AND POLYMYOSITIS

Dermatomyositis (DM) has been linked with underlying malignancy since the publication of 2 case reports of this association in 1916.[4,5] A significantly increased risk of a malignancy among patients with DM has now been established from epidemiologic studies, with the risk of malignancy being highest at the time of or within 1 year of diagnosis.[6] The risk of an underlying malignancy is much lower for polymyositis (PM) but remains statistically significant.

Portions of this article have been adapted from Baer AN, Wortmann RL. The risk of malignancy in patients with dermatomyositis and polymyositis. In: Kagen LJ, editor. The inflammatory myopathies. New York: Humana Press; 2009; with permission.
Division of Rheumatology, Johns Hopkins University School of Medicine, Good Samaritan Hospital, 5200 Eastern Avenue, Mason F. Lord Building Center Tower, Suite 4100, Room 413, Baltimore MD 21224, USA
E-mail address: alanbaer@jhmi.edu

doi:10.1016/j.rdc.2011.01.011
0889-857X/11/$ – see front matter © 2011 Elsevier Inc. All rights reserved.

Epidemiology

The criteria by Bohan and Peter[7] for the diagnosis of PM and DM have been the standard since their publication in 1975, although new criteria are clearly needed.[8] The author identified a total of 35 retrospective case series of inflammatory myopathy in the period between 1975 and 2009 that used these diagnostic criteria and reported the occurrence of malignancy in these patients (**Table 1**). These series from diverse geographic areas include 2326 patients with DM, of whom 557 (24%) had an associated malignancy, and 941 patients with PM, of whom 97 (10%) had an associated malignancy. Carcinomas of the nasopharynx (23%), lung (15%), breast (15%), ovary (8%), colon (5%), stomach (3%), and liver (3%) were the most common malignancies associated with DM.[9,11–16,24,26,30–37,39–41,43–47] There was no predominant tumor type among the limited number of cases associated with PM.

These case series demonstrated that the association with malignancy was much stronger for DM than for PM. These series also highlighted the influence of ethnicity on the types of associated malignancy, the temporal association between the myositis and the malignancy, and the type of evaluation used to recognize the malignancy. These cases were also subject to several forms of bias and thus do not establish a casual link between malignancy and either DM or PM.[48] Almost all cases had a referral bias, using patients seen in tertiary hospitals or specialty clinics. In addition, these cases were subject to Berkson bias; a patient with an occult malignancy who had an associated myopathy was more likely to be hospitalized than a similar patient without myopathy. The bias of increased suspicion and scrutiny for malignancy in patients with PM/DM also existed.

The association of malignancy with DM and PM has been scrutinized in 5 population-based retrospective cohort studies (**Table 2**).[6] In each study, the risk of malignancy in a population-based cohort of patients with PM and DM was compared with that in a normal population. This study design reduced the biases related to referral and diagnostic suspicion of malignancy. In 4 of the studies, all patients with PM and DM hospitalized during a defined period were identified from national hospital discharge databases.[50–53] These studies analyzed cohorts from Sweden, Denmark, Finland, and Scotland, which were ethnically homogeneous. The fifth study identified all cases of biopsy-proven idiopathic inflammatory myopathies in the state of Victoria, Australia during a defined period, using the records of the state reference neuropathology laboratory in which all muscle biopsies results are reviewed.[49] The occurrence of malignancy (excluding nonmelanoma skin cancers) in these patients was determined from national cancer registries and also, in 1 study, from death records for the same period. Malignancies that were identified at the same time or after the diagnosis of myositis were included in the calculation of risk. In some studies, malignancies that were identified during the first 3 to 12 months after the myositis diagnosis were excluded in separate analyses to eliminate diagnostic suspicion bias.[49,51,53]

Each of these 5 studies identified an increased risk of malignancy in patients with DM compared with the general population (see **Table 2**). The overall standardized incidence ratios ranged from 3.8 to 7.7. In addition, 2 of the studies identified an increased but lesser risk in patients with PM, with overall standardized incidence ratios of 1.7 to 2.0.[49,51,52] The cancer risk was increased approximately sixfold during the first year after myositis diagnosis but was lower during the second year, with no significant excess in subsequent years of follow-up.[52] The increased risk of malignancy in DM remained evident when malignancies identified during the first 3 months or the first year after the diagnosis of myositis were excluded.[49,51] Inclusion body myositis was also associated with an increased risk of malignancy in the one study that used muscle biopsy reports for case finding.[49]

These 5 population-based cohort studies have limitations. Of these, 4 studies relied on the accuracy of discharge coding to identify patients with myositis. Airio and colleagues[50] sought to review the medical records of all identified patients and subsequently excluded 226 of 627 patients. Sigurgeirsson and colleagues[53] reviewed every tenth record and found that 7% probably had neither DM nor PM. There was no medical record review in the other 3 studies. With the exception of the study by Buchbinder and colleagues,[49] the diagnoses of PM and DM were based on the criteria by Bohan and Peter[7] in 1975 and thus did not require histopathologic confirmation, which may have led to the misclassification of myositis types and failure to exclude cases of inclusion body myositis from the PM subtype.

Types of Malignancies Associated with DM and PM

The types of malignancies associated with DM and PM in Western countries was best determined by Hill and colleagues[54] with a pooled analysis of the original and more recent follow-up data from the 3 population-based cohort studies performed in Sweden, Denmark, and Finland. Among a total of 618 patients with DM, 115 developed cancer after the diagnosis of myositis. The overall standardized incidence ratio was 3.0 (95% confidence interval [CI], 2.5–3.6). The types of cancer with the greatest increased relative risk were ovary (10.5; 95% CI, 6.1–18.1), lung (5.9; 95% CI, 3.7–9.2), pancreatic (3.8; 95% CI, 1.6–9.0), stomach (3.5; 95% CI, 1.7–7.3), and colorectal (2.5; 95% CI, 1.4–4.4.) cancers and non-Hodgkin lymphoma (3.6; 95% CI, 1.2–11.1). Among 914 patients with PM, 95 developed cancer after the diagnosis of myositis. The relative risks were increased for non-Hodgkin lymphoma (3.7; 95% CI, 1.7–8.2), lung cancer (2.8; 95% CI, 1.8–4.4), and bladder cancer (2.4; 95% CI, 1.3–4.7). The most common cancer type was adenocarcinoma, accounting for 70% of all tumors associated with patients with DM and PM.

Among Asian populations, nasopharyngeal and hepatocellular carcinomas have been strongly associated with DM.[19,35,37,40,47,55] Among 143 patients with probable or definite DM/PM in Taiwan, 18 (13%) had an identified malignancy, the most common being nasopharyngeal carcinoma.[19] Similarly, gastric carcinoma may be the most common associated cancer in Japanese populations.[56]

The histologic type and stage of certain cancers that are associated with DM have been characterized in case reports and series. Ovarian cancer was most often diagnosed during the first year after the diagnosis of DM, almost always epithelial in origin (adenocarcinoma or cystadenocarcinoma) and in Stage III or IV when recognized in the context of DM.[18,57,58] In a review of the literature, Fujita and colleagues[59] identified 24 patients (5 women and 19 men) with primary lung cancer associated with DM or PM. The most common cell types were small cell carcinoma (29%), squamous cell carcinoma (21%), and adenocarcinoma (8%). In 5 of these patients, the onset of myositis preceded the diagnosis of cancer by more than a year.

Clinical Course of Malignancy and Myositis

Isolated case reports have highlighted patients with DM with an associated malignancy in whom the DM improved after successful treatment of the tumor or worsened with evidence of tumor recurrence.[36,60–65] Such a parallel course between the DM and the malignancy is supportive of a paraneoplastic phenomenon but was observed in only 8 of 45 patients reported by Bonnetblanc and colleagues[36] In contrast, Andras and colleagues[12] reported remission of the myositis in 16 of 22 patients with cancer-associated DM who received effective antitumor therapy. The failure to demonstrate this parallel course may reflect the advanced stage of the malignancy when it is

Table 1
Frequency of malignancy in retrospective case series of adult men and women with DM and/or PM (diagnosis established by Bohan and Peter criteria)

References	Malignancy in DM	Malignancy in PM	Source of Patients
9	1/12 (8%)	1/15 (7%)	1 medical center (United States)
10	5/11 (45%)	2/11 (18%)	1 medical center (Canada), 73% fulfilled Bohan and Peter criteria
11	15/40 (38%)	2/35 (6%)	Cases referred to 3 electromyographic laboratories (Singapore)
12	30/103 (29%)	7/206 (3%)	1 medical center (Hungary)
13	10/28 (36%)	2/64 (3%)	1 medical center (Japan)
14	7/27 (26%)	1/31 (3%)	1 medical center (United States)
15	9/20 (45%)	4/15 (27%)	1 medical center (Israel)
16	8/53 (15%)	5/57 (9%)	1 medical center (United States)
17	10/39 (26%)	3/21 (14%)	All general hospitals in Israel, overlap myositis excluded
18	12/56 (21%)	12/84 (14%)	1 medical center (France)
19	16/91 (18%)	2/14 (14%)	1 medical center (Taiwan)
20	9/31 (29%)	8/40 (20%)	1 inpatient rheumatic disease unit (Canada)
21	11/50 (22%)	18/65 (28%)	1 medical center (United States)
22	7/36 (19%)	9/69 (13%)	1 medical center (Australia)
23	3/19 (16%)	4/51 (8%)	Multiple medical centers (Sweden)
24	4/10 (40%)	0/18	Muscle biopsy cases in 1 laboratory (Canada)
25	7/39 (18%)	2/20 (10%)	1 medical center (France)
26	5/16 (31%)	6/25 (24%)	1 medical center (Korea)
27	13/33 (39%)	3/7 (43%)	1 medical center (France)
28	3/24 (13%)	3/34 (9%)	1 inpatient rheumatic disease unit (United States)
29	25/62 (40%)	3/59 (5%)	1 medical center (United States)
30	12/50 (24%)	—	1 medical center (Bulgaria)
31	9/32 (28%)	—	1 medical center (France)
32	13/32 (41%)	—	1 medical center (France)
33	23/53 (43%)	—	2 medical centers (United Kingdom)
34	6/10 (60%)	—	1 medical center (Singapore)
35	12/38 (32%)	—	1 medical center (Singapore)
36	34/118 (28%)	—	All dermatologic university medical centers in France
37	12/28 (43%)	—	1 medical center (Singapore)
38	9/18 (50%)	—	1 medical center (Norway)
39	20/130 (15%)	—	All university hospitals of Tunisia
40	5/12 (41%)	—	1 medical center (Singapore)
41	9/18 (50%)	—	1 medical center (Denmark)
42	16/84 (19%)	—	1 medical center (Hungary)

(continued on next page)

Table 1 (*continued*)			
References	**Malignancy in DM**	**Malignancy in PM**	**Source of Patients**
43	10/29 (35%)	—	1 medical center (France)
44	5/43 (12%)	—	1 medical center (United States)
45	29/121	—	2 medical centers (France)
46	8/32	—	1 medical center (Bosnia)
47	115/678	—	1 medical center (China)

Data from Bohan A, Peter JB. Polymyositis and dermatomyositis (first of two parts). N Engl J Med 1975;292(7):344–7; *Adapted from* Baer AN, Wortmann RL. The risk of malignancy in patients with dermatomyositis and polymyositis. In: Kagen LJ, editor. The inflammatory myopathies. New York: Humana Press; 2009. p. 309; with permission.

ultimately diagnosed.[66] The excess risk of malignancy that remains as long as 5 years after the diagnosis of myositis needs further study because it challenges the concept of a paraneoplastic phenomenon.[49]

Risk Factors for Malignancy in DM and PM

A variety of factors influence the risk of an associated malignancy in DM/PM (**Box 1**). The risk of malignancy is higher in older patients with DM or PM. In the population-based cohort studies by Airio and colleagues[50] and Chow and colleagues,[52] an increased risk of malignancy was only evident in patients older than 45 to 50 years at the time of myositis diagnosis. An increased risk was evident for patients with DM aged 45 to 74 years and patients with PM aged 15 to 44 years in the study by Stockton and colleagues.[51] This increased risk of malignancy in older patients with DM was also evident in other cohort analyses[19,20,45,54] but not in 2 others.[21,67]

Gender is not a consistent risk factor for malignancy in patients with DM. Standardized incidence ratios were higher for men in the studies by Airio and colleagues[50] and Stockton and colleagues[51] but not in the study by Sigurgeirsson and colleagues[53] An increased risk of malignancy in patients with PM was evident for women but not for men in the study by Stockton and colleagues.[51]

Table 2 Population-based cohort studies of the association of malignancy with DM and PM				
References	**Frequency of Malignancy in DM**	**DM SIR**	**Frequency of Malignancy in PM**	**PM SIR**
49	36/85 (42%)	6.2 (3.9–10.0)	58/321 (18%)	2.0 (1.4–2.7)
50	19/71 (27%)	6.5 (3.9–10.0)	12/175 (7%)	1.0 (0.5–1.8)
51	77/286 (27%)	7.7 (5.7–10.1)	71/419 (17%)	2.1 (1.5–2.9)
52	31/203 (15%)	3.8 (2.6–5.4)	26/336 (8%)	1.7 (1.1–2.4)
53	59/392 (15%)	2.4 (1.6–3.6), men; 3.4 (2.4–4.7), women	37/396 (9%)	1.8 (1.1–2.7), men; 1.7 (1.0–2.5), women

Abbreviation: SIR, standardized incidence ratio.

Reproduced from Baer AN, Wortmann RL. The risk of malignancy in patients with dermatomyositis and polymyositis. In: Kagen LJ, editor. The inflammatory myopathies. New York: Humana Press; 2009. p. 309; with permission.

Box 1
Risk factors for underlying malignancy in myositis

Increased risk

Host factors

- Older age at onset[11,12,19,45,51,54,68]

More severe skin disease

- Cutaneous necrosis and ulceration[12,31,32,45,46,69,70]
- Leukocytoclastic vasculitis[32,71]
- Resistance to therapy[12,31,35,42]

More severe muscle disease

- Distal muscle weakness[12,42]
- Dysphagia[12,38]
- Respiratory muscle involvement[12]
- Refractory to treatment[12]

Laboratory markers

- Elevated erythrocyte sedimentation ratio and C-reactive protein level[32,41,43,72]
- Low C4 level[45]
- Lower serum albumin level[43]
- Elevated levels of tumor markers[12,73–75]

Decreased risk

Overlap features

- Interstitial lung disease[12,19,29,42]
- Arthritis/arthralgia[12]
- Raynaud phenomenon[12]
- Cardiac involvement[12]
- Fever[12]
- Positive test results for antinuclear antibodies and extractable nuclear antigens[12,29,42]
- Jo-1 antibodies[12]
- Lymphopenia[45]

Specific features of the DM rash are predictive of underlying malignancy, including the presence of cutaneous necrosis and ulceration,[12,31,32,45,46,69,70] periungual erythema,[45] and leukocytoclastic vasculitis.[32,71] Malignant erythema, a fiery red suffusion on the face, scalp, neck, and shoulders, has been reported to be more common in patients with DM with an underlying malignancy.[76] The rash may be more refractory to treatment.[35,42]

Myositis has been reported to be more severe in the setting of an underlying malignancy, with a higher frequency of distal muscle weakness,[12,42] dysphagia,[12,38] respiratory muscle involvement,[12] and resistance to immunosuppressive treatment.[12] These findings have not been confirmed by other investigators.[21] In addition, amyopathic DM has also been observed in this setting.[37,77,78]

The presence of clinical or laboratory features that overlap with other connective tissue diseases diminishes the risk of an underlying malignancy. These features include the presence of interstitial lung disease,[12,19,42] arthritis,[12] Raynaud phenomenon,[12] fever,[12] and a high titer of antinuclear antibodies.[12,42] On the other hand, an increased risk of underlying malignancy was evident for myositis associated with connective tissue disease in the epidemiologic study by Buchbinder and colleagues,[49] but the numbers were too small to make this a definitive association.

Myositis-specific antibodies, such as Jo-1, are markers of specific subsets of the idiopathic inflammatory myopathies but can also be seen in up to 13% of cases of cancer-associated myositis (**Table 3**). The presence of these antibodies does not preclude the diagnosis of cancer-related myositis.[83] Kaji and colleagues[84] identified a novel autoantibody reactive with 155- and 140-kDa nuclear proteins (155/140 antibody) in patients with DM. This autoantibody was present in 71% of patients with DM with an underlying malignancy and in only 11% of those without malignancy. In a study by Chinoy and colleagues,[79] this 155/140 antibody had a sensitivity of 50% and a specificity of 96% for cancer-associated myositis. When combined with negative results of hospital-based routine testing for Jo-1, Ku, PM-Scl, U1-RNP, and U3-RNP antibodies, a positive 155/140 antibody result had a sensitivity of 94% and a negative predictive value of 99%.

Certain laboratory markers in patients with DM or PM may also serve as predictors of an underlying malignancy. The erythrocyte sedimentation rate and C-reactive protein are typically higher in the setting of an underlying malignancy.[32,41,72] The maximal level of creatine kinase (CK) has been reported to be lower in patients with DM/PM with an underlying malignancy than in those with DM/PM without an underlying malignancy.[12,26,42,85] However, this observation is not uniform.[21,27,46] Tumor marker elevation is associated with an increased risk of developing an underlying malignancy.[12,73–75] However, the sensitivity of cancer antigen (CA) 125 elevation for detecting ovarian cancer in patients with DM was only 50% in the study by Whitmore and colleagues.[75]

Evaluation for Malignancy

All patients presenting with an inflammatory myopathy, regardless of their age or myositis type, should undergo a careful history taking and physical examination as well as routine screening laboratory tests. Tumor marker screening (eg, α-fetoprotein, carcinoembryonic antigen, CA 125, prostate-specific antigen, and CA 19–9) and radiographies (eg, chest radiography and mammography) appropriate to the age, gender,

Table 3
Myositis-specific antibodies in cancer-associated myositis and idiopathic myositis

References	Number of Patients	MSA in CAM	MSA in Non-CAM
79	282	3/16	92/266
80	97	1/3	38/94
81	86	2/8	26/78
82	556	4/51	195/505
Total	842	10/78 (13%)	351/943 (37%)

Abbreviations: CAM, cancer-associated myositis; MSA, myositis-specific antibodies.

Reproduced from Baer AN, Wortmann RL. The risk of malignancy in patients with dermatomyositis and polymyositis. In: Kagen LJ, editor. The inflammatory myopathies. New York: Humana Press; 2009. p. 312; with permission.

and ethnicity of the patient are also prudent.[14,33,73,86] This evaluation should include an examination of the testes in men, breast and pelvis in women, and rectum in all patients. Fecal occult blood testing and colonoscopy should be performed in all patients older than 50 years and in younger patients with strong risk factors for colorectal cancer.[87] Any abnormalities detected on this initial screening evaluation should be pursued carefully. Because the risk of an underlying malignancy is much higher in patients with DM, a more extensive evaluation for malignancy is advisable in specific subsets of these patients. A woman with a new diagnosis of DM should undergo thorough gynecologic examination to screen for an ovarian carcinoma. This evaluation should include pelvic and transvaginal ultrasonography, measurement of CA 125, and, if necessary, pelvic computed tomography.[18,58,66] A repeat evaluation at 3 and 6 months has also been recommended in women presenting with DM whose initial evaluation for ovarian cancer was negative.[18] This recommendation is predicated on the fact that ovarian malignancies have a strong association with DM and may not be detected with a routine pelvic examination. The type of malignancy evaluation performed for DM should be modified for specific ethnic groups in which specific types of cancers are overrepresented. Patients with DM of Chinese descent need to be evaluated for nasopharyngeal and hepatocellular carcinomas and those of Japanese descent should be evaluated for gastric carcinoma.[19,35,37,40,55,56]

The vigor with which the search for an underlying malignancy is pursued in patients with DM has been contested, particularly as the diagnostic tools, such as positron emission tomography, have become more sensitive, yet also unacceptably expensive when used indiscriminately.[88] Although most malignancies can be identified with the screening evaluation detailed earlier, some are missed and do not become clinically apparent until later in the patient's clinical course.[89] The malignancies that are most likely to be missed by screening examinations include ovarian, pancreatic, and lung cancers and lymphoma. Accordingly, computed tomographic (CT) imaging of the chest, abdomen, and pelvis is prudent in the subset of patients with new-onset DM who are older or who have risk factors for specific types of malignancy (family history of ovarian cancer, smokers). The use of diagnostic tools for malignancy that go beyond the screening measures described earlier should be considered in patients with DM with a more severe rash that is associated with cutaneous necrosis[32,69,70] or severe muscle disease that is refractory to steroid therapy.[12,42,49] In addition, a recurrence of the rash or muscle weakness after initial successful treatment should prompt a second look for malignancy. This type of evaluation may not be necessary in patients whose myositis is clearly associated with another connective tissue disease, such as lupus or scleroderma.

Pathogenesis

The association between DM/PM and a malignancy has several potential biologic explanations, including the presence of common host predispositions, infectious triggers, toxic exposures, or the presence of a paraneoplastic syndrome. The confluence of DM and cancer, with both diagnoses often being established within 1 year of each other, supports the presence of a paraneoplastic syndrome. The leading hypothesis to explain this relationship is an immune reaction to the tumor that cross-reacts with antigens in skin and muscle, leading to DM. Such an immune reaction occurs in autoimmune paraneoplastic neurologic disorders in which immune-mediated neuronal damage develops in the setting of solid tumors of the breast, ovary, and lung.[90] Casciola-Rosen and colleagues[91] observed that the myositis autoantigens, Mi-2 and histidyl transfer RNA synthetase, are expressed at high levels in myositis muscles, particularly in regenerating muscle fibers, as well as in adenocarcinomas of the lung and breast but not in the corresponding normal tissues. These observations thus identify regenerating muscle cells and certain tumors as the source of ongoing myositis autoantigen expression in myositis. These investigators have proposed a model of crossover immunity in which an initial cellular immune response is directed at tumor cells overexpressing antigens commonly targeted in myositis. In the setting of muscle injury and regeneration, myositis-specific autoantigens are expressed. An immune reaction initially directed at these autoantigens expressed in tumor cells crosses over and leads to the development of myositis.

NECROTIZING MYOPATHY

A necrotizing myopathy can develop in patients with an underlying malignancy.[92,93] These patients develop severe weakness over a period of 1 to 3 months, with predominant involvement of the proximal musculature. Serum CK levels are elevated, often to very high levels. Muscle fiber necrosis in the absence of mononuclear cell infiltrates is the primary histopathologic feature. Emslie-Smith and Engel[94] described a distinctive microangiopathy with thick pipestem capillaries and microvascular deposits of complement membrane attack complex in 3 such patients (one of whom had a carcinoma). The most commonly associated malignancies include adenocarcinomas of the gastrointestinal tract and prostate, transitional cell carcinoma of the bladder, breast carcinomas, and non–small cell lung cancer.[93,95] Necrotizing myopathies may also be seen in certain forms of drug-induced myotoxicity, such as myopathies associated with signal recognition particle antibodies and 200/100-kDa antibodies, associated with Behçet disease, and occasionally in patients with PM as a result of a sampling error.[96–98] Prolonged high-dose prednisone therapy with or without intravenous immunoglobulin may result in the return of normal or near-normal muscle strength.[92,99]

EATON-LAMBERT SYNDROME

Eaton-Lambert syndrome is a rare disorder of neuromuscular junction transmission, arising from IgG antibodies that block voltage-gated calcium channels on presynaptic cholinergic nerve terminals. Approximately 50% of patients with this disorder have an underlying malignancy, usually small cell lung cancer. In the remaining patients, there may be other findings indicating an autoimmune disorder, such as vitiligo, pernicious anemia, and thyroid disease. Most patients are older than 40 years at presentation. Affected patients generally present with the insidious onset of hip girdle weakness, resulting in a waddling gait. Weakness of the proximal upper limbs is evident as the disease progresses but remains less severe than that of the lower extremities. Tenderness of the weak muscles may be present. Patients may report increased weakness and/or muscle fatigue, aching, and stiffness after prolonged exercise. Autonomic symptoms are often present, including dry mouth, dry eyes, impotence, orthostatic hypotension, and constipation. Ocular and bulbar muscle involvement is rare and never presents on initial presentation, a feature that distinguishes this disease from myasthenia gravis (MG). On examination, patients may exhibit a progressive increase in strength during the first few seconds of sustained maximum effort, whereas continued testing leads to fatigue and increasing weakness. Absent or reduced tendon reflexes, ptosis, neck flexor weakness, and a sluggish pupillary reaction to light are additional findings.

Electromyographic studies show characteristic abnormalities, including low-amplitude compound muscle action potentials on motor nerve stimulation, which increase by more than 100% in amplitude after high-frequency repetitive nerve stimulation. Antibodies to voltage-gated calcium channels are present in nearly all patients with an associated malignancy and in more than 90% of those without.

The diagnosis of Eaton-Lambert syndrome should prompt an aggressive evaluation for malignancy. Effective treatment of the cancer often improves the symptoms and signs of Eaton-Lambert syndrome. The drug 3,4-diaminopyridine may lead to improvement in strength. This drug blocks potassium channels, preventing repolarization of the nerve terminal, and thereby allows more calcium entry into the cell, which in turn increases the release of acetylcholine. Immunosuppressive therapy with corticosteroids or azathioprine is often used for patients with an anticipated need for long-term therapy, usually those in whom the Eaton-Lambert syndrome is occurring in the absence of an underlying malignancy. Intravenous immunoglobulin and plasma exchange may be used for severe disease or for those who cannot tolerate immunosuppressive therapy.

MG

MG is a disorder of neuromuscular transmission that arises from antibodies that bind the acetylcholine receptor on the postsynaptic membrane of the neuromuscular junction. The cardinal symptoms are muscular weakness and fatigability, particularly later in the day or with prolonged exertion. MG is associated with a thymoma in 10% to 15% of patients, and this concurrence is considered to be a paraneoplastic phenomenon. MG occurs in association with extrathymic malignancies but not at a frequency higher than that in age- and sex-matched controls.[100] Paraneoplastic MG affects both genders equally and can occur at any age but has a peak age of onset of approximately 50 years. Virtually all patients with paraneoplastic MG have antiacetylcholine receptor antibodies. In contrast to other forms of MG, most patients with paraneoplastic MG also have antibodies to titin and ryanodine. In one study, these antibodies were found, respectively, in 95% and 70% of paraneoplastic MG, 10% and 0% of early-onset MG, and 58% and 14% of late-onset MG.[101] The detection of antibodies to ryanodine provided a specificity and sensitivity 70% for the diagnosis of paraneoplastic MG.[101] Patients with MG with antiryanodine antibodies, many of whom have an associated thymoma, differ from patients with early-onset MG in their clinical features, having more frequent involvement of their neck muscles and sparing of their limb muscles at disease onset.

All patients with MG need to be evaluated with an anterior mediastinum CT or magnetic resonance imaging to examine for thymoma. If detected, the thymoma should be removed surgically to avoid the risk of tumor invasion and to affect favorably the natural course of the disease. Paraneoplastic MG usually persists after thymectomy and requires long-term therapy with acetylcholinesterase inhibitors, often in combination with immunosuppressive agents. The prognosis of paraneoplastic MG is comparable with that in age-matched patients with MG without a history of thymoma.

STIFF PERSON SYNDROME

Stiff person syndrome is a rare autoimmune neuromuscular disorder characterized by stiffness and rigidity of the axial and proximal limb muscles. Paraspinal and abdominal muscle rigidity typically leads to a rigid posture with an exaggerated lumbar lordosis. A cardinal feature of the syndrome is muscle spasms precipitated by touch, involuntary movement, emotional stress, and unexpected loud noises. The sudden provocation of muscle spasms may result in the patient losing balance and falling to the ground in a statuelike stance because of the failure of normal righting responses.

Electromyography findings demonstrate continuous motor unit activity in affected muscles, eliminated by the administration of diazepam and other benzodiazepines. Stiff person syndrome has both nonparaneoplastic and paraneoplastic variants. The former is associated with high titers of antibodies to glutamic acid decarboxylase (GAD). Many of these patients have other autoimmune diseases, particularly diabetes mellitus type 1, and also thyroiditis, vitiligo, and pernicious anemia. The paraneoplastic variant is associated with antibodies to amphiphysin and occurs primarily in association with breast adenocarcinoma and small cell lung carcinoma. This variant may develop before the recognition of breast cancer and is characterized by less severe lumbar lordosis and more prominent arm and neck involvement than the nonparaneoplastic variant. The nonparaneoplastic variant of stiff person syndrome associated with GAD antibodies is responsive to intravenous immunoglobulin. The paraneoplastic variant responds to treatment of the malignancy; some patients may benefit from plasmapheresis and corticosteroids.

SUMMARY

There are 2 important clinical implications of paraneoplastic muscle disease. First, muscle weakness or other dysfunction that arises in the setting of a known malignancy needs to be evaluated thoroughly. A variety of pathogenetic mechanisms may be applicable, including paraneoplastic phenomena. Approaches to the treatment of the associated muscle disease thus depend on this careful evaluation. Paraneoplastic muscle disease is amenable to therapy, ranging from surgical or medical treatment of the malignancy to the use of immunosuppressive agents. Second, the occurrence of certain forms of muscle disease, particularly myositis and disorders of neuromuscular transmission, requires a vigilant search for an underlying malignancy.

The most common paraneoplastic muscle disease is DM. Most malignancies associated with DM are adenocarcinomas, particularly of the ovary, lung, pancreas, stomach, and colon. Nasopharyngeal carcinoma is commonly associated with DM in Asian countries. A search for an underlying malignancy is important in patients presenting with DM or PM, although the scope and vigor of this evaluation needs to be tailored to the individual patient, taking into account the presence of factors that may increase or diminish the likelihood of an associated malignancy.

REFERENCES

1. Honnorat J, Antoine JC. Paraneoplastic neurological syndromes. Orphanet J Rare Dis 2007;2:22.
2. Darnell RB, Posner JB. Paraneoplastic syndromes involving the nervous system. N Engl J Med 2003;349(16):1543–54.
3. Graus F, Delattre JY, Antoine JC, et al. Recommended diagnostic criteria for paraneoplastic neurological syndromes. J Neurol Neurosurg Psychiatry 2004;75(8): 1135–40.
4. Stertz G. Polymyositis. Berl Klin Wochenschr 1916;53:489.
5. Kankeleit H. Uber primare nichteitrige polymyositis. Dtsch Arch Klin Med 1916; 120:335–49 [in German].
6. Buchbinder R, Hill CL. Malignancy in patients with inflammatory myopathy. Curr Rheumatol Rep 2002;4(5):415–26.
7. Bohan A, Peter JB. Polymyositis and dermatomyositis (first of two parts). N Engl J Med 1975;292(7):344–7.
8. Miller FW, Rider LG, Plotz PH, et al. Diagnostic criteria for polymyositis and dermatomyositis. Lancet 2003;362(9397):1762–3 [author reply: 1763].

9. Hoffman GS, Franck WA, Raddatz DA, et al. Presentation, treatment, and prognosis of idiopathic inflammatory muscle disease in a rural hospital. Am J Med 1983;75(3):433–8.

10. Baron M, Small P. Polymyositis/dermatomyositis: clinical features and outcome in 22 patients. J Rheumatol 1985;12(2):283–6.

11. Koh ET, Seow A, Ong B, et al. Adult onset polymyositis/dermatomyositis: clinical and laboratory features and treatment response in 75 patients. Ann Rheum Dis 1993;52(12):857–61.

12. Andras C, Ponyi A, Constantin T, et al. Dermatomyositis and polymyositis associated with malignancy: a 21-year retrospective study. J Rheumatol 2008;35(3):438–44.

13. Wakata N, Kurihara T, Saito E, et al. Polymyositis and dermatomyositis associated with malignancy: a 30-year retrospective study. Int J Dermatol 2002;41(11):729–34.

14. Callen JP, Hyla JF, Bole GG Jr, et al. The relationship of dermatomyositis and polymyositis to internal malignancy. Arch Dermatol 1980;116(3):295–8.

15. Maoz CR, Langevitz P, Livneh A, et al. High incidence of malignancies in patients with dermatomyositis and polymyositis: an 11-year analysis. Semin Arthritis Rheum 1998;27(5):319–24.

16. Bohan A, Peter JB, Bowman RL, et al. Computer-assisted analysis of 153 patients with polymyositis and dermatomyositis. Medicine (Baltimore) 1977;56(4):255–86.

17. Benbassat J, Gefel D, Larholt K, et al. Prognostic factors in polymyositis/dermatomyositis. A computer-assisted analysis of ninety-two cases. Arthritis Rheum 1985;28(3):249–55.

18. Cherin P, Piette JC, Herson S, et al. Dermatomyositis and ovarian cancer: a report of 7 cases and literature review. J Rheumatol 1993;20(11):1897–9.

19. Chen YJ, Wu CY, Shen JL. Predicting factors of malignancy in dermatomyositis and polymyositis: a case-control study. Br J Dermatol 2001;144(4):825–31.

20. Manchul LA, Jin A, Pritchard KI, et al. The frequency of malignant neoplasms in patients with polymyositis-dermatomyositis. A controlled study. Arch Intern Med 1985;145(10):1835–9.

21. Lakhanpal S, Bunch TW, Ilstrup DM, et al. Polymyositis-dermatomyositis and malignant lesions: does an association exist? Mayo Clin Proc 1986;61(8):645–53.

22. Tymms KE, Webb J. Dermatopolymyositis and other connective tissue diseases: a review of 105 cases. J Rheumatol 1985;12(6):1140–8.

23. Henriksson KG, Sandstedt P. Polymyositis—treatment and prognosis. A study of 107 patients. Acta Neurol Scand 1982;65(4):280–300.

24. Holden DJ, Brownell AK, Fritzler MJ. Clinical and serologic features of patients with polymyositis or dermatomyositis. Can Med Assoc J 1985;132(6):649–53.

25. Ponge A, Mussini JM, Ponge T, et al. Paraneoplastic dermatopolymyositis. Rev Med Interne 1987;8(3):251–6.

26. Lee SW, Jung SY, Park MC, et al. Malignancies in Korean patients with inflammatory myopathy. Yonsei Med J 2006;47(4):519–23.

27. Sparsa A, Liozon E, Herrmann F, et al. Routine vs extensive malignancy search for adult dermatomyositis and polymyositis: a study of 40 patients. Arch Dermatol 2002;138(7):885–90.

28. Hochberg MC, Feldman D, Stevens MB. Adult onset polymyositis/dermatomyositis: an analysis of clinical and laboratory features and survival in 76 patients with a review of the literature. Semin Arthritis Rheum 1986;15(3):168–78.

29. Antiochos BB, Brown LA, Wortmann RL, et al. Malignancy is associated with dermatomyositis, but not polymyositis in northern New England. Arthritis Rheum 2008;58(Suppl 9):S230–1.
30. Dourmishev LA. Dermatomyositis associated with malignancy. 12 case reports. Adv Exp Med Biol 1999;455:193–9.
31. Gallais V, Crickx B, Belaich S. Prognostic factors and predictive signs of malignancy in adult dermatomyositis. Ann Dermatol Venereol 1996;123(11):722–6.
32. Basset-Seguin N, Roujeau JC, Gherardi R, et al. Prognostic factors and predictive signs of malignancy in adult dermatomyositis. A study of 32 cases. Arch Dermatol 1990;126(5):633–7.
33. Cox NH, Lawrence CM, Langtry JA, et al. Disease associations and an evaluation of screening investigations for malignancy. Arch Dermatol 1990;126(1):61–5.
34. Goh CL, Rajan VS. Dermatomyositis in a skin clinic. Ann Acad Med Singapore 1983;12(1):6–12.
35. Leow YH, Goh CL. Malignancy in adult dermatomyositis. Int J Dermatol 1997; 36(12):904–7.
36. Bonnetblanc JM, Bernard P, Fayol J. Dermatomyositis and malignancy. A multicenter cooperative study. Dermatologica 1990;180(4):212–6.
37. Ang P, Sugeng MW, Chua SH. Classical and amyopathic dermatomyositis seen at the National Skin Centre of Singapore: a 3-year retrospective review of their clinical characteristics and association with malignancy. Ann Acad Med Singapore 2000;29(2):219–23.
38. Selvaag E, Thune P, Austad J. Dermatomyositis and cancer. A retrospective study. Tidsskr Nor Laegeforen 1994;114(20):2378–80.
39. Mebazaa A, Boussen H, Nouira R, et al. Dermatomyositis and malignancy in Tunisia: a multicenter national retrospective study of 20 cases. J Am Acad Dermatol 2003;48(4):530–4.
40. Chan HL. Dermatomyositis and cancer in Singapore. Int J Dermatol 1985;24(7): 447–50.
41. Vesterager L, Worm AM, Thomsen K. Dermatomyositis and malignancy. Clin Exp Dermatol 1980;5(1):31–5.
42. Ponyi A, Constantin T, Garami M, et al. Cancer-associated myositis: clinical features and prognostic signs. Ann N Y Acad Sci 2005;1051:64–71.
43. Rose C, Hatron PY, Brouillard M, et al. Predictive signs of cancers in dermatomyositis. Study of 29 cases. Rev Med Interne 1994;15(1):19–24.
44. Dawkins MA, Jorizzo JL, Walker FO, et al. Dermatomyositis: a dermatology-based case series. J Am Acad Dermatol 1998;38(3):397–404.
45. Fardet L, Dupuy A, Gain M, et al. Factors associated with underlying malignancy in a retrospective cohort of 121 patients with dermatomyositis. Medicine (Baltimore) 2009;88(2):91–7.
46. Prohic A, Kasumagic-Halilovic E, Simic D, et al. Clinical and biological factors predictive of malignancy in dermatomyositis. J Eur Acad Dermatol Venereol 2009;23(5):591–2.
47. Zhang W, Jiang SP, Huang L. Dermatomyositis and malignancy: a retrospective study of 115 cases. Eur Rev Med Pharmacol Sci 2009;13(2):77–80.
48. Masi AT, Hochberg MC. Temporal association of polymyositis-dermatomyositis with malignancy: methodologic and clinical considerations. Mt Sinai J Med 1988;55(6):471–8.
49. Buchbinder R, Forbes A, Hall S, et al. Incidence of malignant disease in biopsy-proven inflammatory myopathy. A population-based cohort study. Ann Intern Med 2001;134(12):1087–95.

50. Airio A, Pukkala E, Isomaki H. Elevated cancer incidence in patients with derma-tomyositis: a population based study. J Rheumatol 1995;22(7):1300–3.

51. Stockton D, Doherty VR, Brewster DH. Risk of cancer in patients with dermato-myositis or polymyositis, and follow-up implications: a Scottish population-based cohort study. Br J Cancer 2001;85(1):41–5.

52. Chow WH, Gridley G, Mellemkjaer L, et al. Cancer risk following polymyositis and dermatomyositis: a nationwide cohort study in Denmark. Cancer Causes Control 1995;6(1):9–13.

53. Sigurgeirsson B, Lindelof B, Edhag O, et al. Risk of cancer in patients with der-matomyositis or polymyositis. A population-based study. N Engl J Med 1992; 326(6):363–7.

54. Hill CL, Zhang Y, Sigurgeirsson B, et al. Frequency of specific cancer types in dermatomyositis and polymyositis: a population-based study. Lancet 2001; 357(9250):96–100.

55. Peng JC, Sheen TS, Hsu MM. Nasopharyngeal carcinoma with dermatomyosi-tis. Analysis of 12 cases. Arch Otolaryngol Head Neck Surg 1995;121(11): 1298–301.

56. Hatada T, Aoki I, Ikeda H, et al. Dermatomyositis and malignancy: case report and review of the Japanese literature. Tumori 1996;82(3):273–5.

57. Davis MD, Ahmed I. Ovarian malignancy in patients with dermatomyositis and polymyositis: a retrospective analysis of fourteen cases. J Am Acad Dermatol 1997;37(5 Pt 1):730–3.

58. Mordel N, Margalioth EJ, Harats N, et al. Concurrence of ovarian cancer and dermatomyositis. A report of two cases and literature review. J Reprod Med 1988;33(7):649–55.

59. Fujita J, Tokuda M, Bandoh S, et al. Primary lung cancer associated with poly-myositis/dermatomyositis, with a review of the literature. Rheumatol Int 2001; 20(2):81–4.

60. Masuda H, Urushibara M, Kihara K. Successful treatment of dermatomyositis associated with adenocarcinoma of the prostate after radical prostatectomy. J Urol 2003;169(3):1084.

61. Tallai B, Flasko T, Gyorgy T, et al. Prostate cancer underlying acute, definitive dermatomyositis: successful treatment with radical perineal prostatectomy. Clin Rheumatol 2006;25(1):119–20.

62. Yoshinaga A, Hayashi T, Ishii N, et al. Successful cure of dermatomyositis after treatment of nonseminomatous testicular cancer. Int J Urol 2005;12(6):593–5.

63. Solomon SD, Maurer KH. Association of dermatomyositis and dysgerminoma in a 16-year-old patient. Arthritis Rheum 1983;26(4):572–3.

64. Callen JP. Dermatomyositis and female malignancy. J Surg Oncol 1986;32(2):121–4.

65. Barnes BE, Mawr B. Dermatomyositis and malignancy. A review of the literature. Ann Intern Med 1976;84(1):68–76.

66. Whitmore SE, Rosenshein NB, Provost TT. Ovarian cancer in patients with der-matomyositis. Medicine (Baltimore) 1994;73(3):153–60.

67. Pautas E, Cherin P, Piette JC, et al. Features of polymyositis and dermatomyo-sitis in the elderly: a case-control study. Clin Exp Rheumatol 2000;18(2):241–4.

68. Marie I, Hatron PY, Levesque H, et al. Influence of age on characteristics of pol-ymyositis and dermatomyositis in adults. Medicine (Baltimore) 1999;78(3): 139–47.

69. Mahe E, Descamps V, Burnouf M, et al. A helpful clinical sign predictive of cancer in adult dermatomyositis: cutaneous necrosis. Arch Dermatol 2003; 139(4):539.

70. Mautner GH, Grossman ME, Silvers DN, et al. Epidermal necrosis as a predictive sign of malignancy in adult dermatomyositis. Cutis 1998;61(4):190–4.
71. Hunger RE, Durr C, Brand CU. Cutaneous leukocytoclastic vasculitis in derma-tomyositis suggests malignancy. Dermatology 2001;202(2):123–6.
72. Amerio P, Girardelli CR, Proietto G, et al. Usefulness of erythrocyte sedimenta-tion rate as tumor marker in cancer associated dermatomyositis. Eur J Dermatol 2002;12(2):165–9.
73. Amoura Z, Duhaut P, Huong DL, et al. Tumor antigen markers for the detection of solid cancers in inflammatory myopathies. Cancer Epidemiol Biomarkers Prev 2005;14(5):1279–82.
74. O'Gradaigh D, Merry P. Tumour markers in dermatomyositis: useful or useless? Br J Rheumatol 1998;37(8):914.
75. Whitmore SE, Anhalt GJ, Provost TT, et al. Serum CA-125 screening for ovarian cancer in patients with dermatomyositis. Gynecol Oncol 1997;65(2):241–4.
76. Winkelmann RK. The cutaneous diagnosis of dermatomyositis, lupus erythema-tosus, and scleroderma. N Y State J Med 1963;63:3080–6.
77. Whitmore SE, Watson R, Rosenshein NB, et al. Dermatomyositis sine myositis: association with malignancy. J Rheumatol 1996;23(1):101–5.
78. Fung WK, Chan HL, Lam WM. Amyopathic dermatomyositis in Hong Kong—association with nasopharyngeal carcinoma. Int J Dermatol 1998;37(9):659–63.
79. Chinoy H, Fertig N, Oddis CV, et al. The diagnostic utility of myositis autoanti-body testing for predicting the risk of cancer-associated myositis. Ann Rheum Dis 2007;66(10):1345–9.
80. Hengstman GJ, Brouwer R, Egberts WT, et al. Clinical and serological charac-teristics of 125 Dutch myositis patients. Myositis specific autoantibodies aid in the differential diagnosis of the idiopathic inflammatory myopathies. J Neurol 2002;249(1):69–75.
81. Selva-O'Callaghan A, Labrador-Horrillo M, Solans-Laque R, et al. Myositis-specific and myositis-associated antibodies in a series of eighty-eight Mediter-ranean patients with idiopathic inflammatory myopathy. Arthritis Rheum 2006; 55(5):791–8.
82. O'Hanlon TP, Carrick DM, Targoff IN, et al. Immunogenetic risk and protective factors for the idiopathic inflammatory myopathies: distinct HLA-A, -B, -Cw, -DRB1, and -DQA1 allelic profiles distinguish European American patients with different myositis autoantibodies. Medicine (Baltimore) 2006;85(2): 111–27.
83. Legault D, McDermott J, Crous-Tsanaclis AM, et al. Cancer-associated myositis in the presence of anti-Jo1 autoantibodies and the antisynthetase syndrome. J Rheumatol 2008;35(1):169–71.
84. Kaji K, Fujimoto M, Hasegawa M, et al. Identification of a novel autoantibody reactive with 155 and 140 kDa nuclear proteins in patients with dermatomyositis: an association with malignancy. Rheumatology (Oxford) 2007;46(1):25–8.
85. Fudman EJ, Schnitzer TJ. Dermatomyositis without creatine kinase elevation. A poor prognostic sign. Am J Med 1986;80(2):329–32.
86. Callen JP. The value of malignancy evaluation in patients with dermatomyositis. J Am Acad Dermatol 1982;6(2):253–9.
87. Pautas E, Cherin P. Investigation of polymyositis-dermatomyositis in older people should include rectal examination. J Am Geriatr Soc 1998;46(12):1584.
88. Callen JP. When and how should the patient with dermatomyositis or amyo-pathic dermatomyositis be assessed for possible cancer? Arch Dermatol 2002;138(7):969–71.

89. Schulman P, Kerr LD, Spiera H. A reexamination of the relationship between myositis and malignancy. J Rheumatol 1991;18(11):1689–92.

90. Levine SM. Cancer and myositis: new insights into an old association. Curr Opin Rheumatol 2006;18(6):620–4.

91. Casciola-Rosen L, Nagaraju K, Plotz P, et al. Enhanced autoantigen expression in regenerating muscle cells in idiopathic inflammatory myopathy. J Exp Med 2005;201(4):591–601.

92. Bronner IM, Hoogendijk JE, Wintzen AR, et al. Necrotising myopathy, an unusual presentation of a steroid-responsive myopathy. J Neurol 2003;250(4):480–5.

93. Levin MI, Mozaffar T, Al-Lozi MT, et al. Paraneoplastic necrotizing myopathy: clinical and pathological features. Neurology 1998;50(3):764–7.

94. Emslie-Smith AM, Engel AG. Necrotizing myopathy with pipestem capillaries, microvascular deposition of the complement membrane attack complex (MAC), and minimal cellular infiltration. Neurology 1991;41(6):936–9.

95. Silvestre J, Santos L, Batalha V, et al. Paraneoplastic necrotizing myopathy in a woman with breast cancer: a case report. J Med Case Reports 2009;3:95.

96. Hengstman GJ, ter Laak HJ, Vree Egberts WT, et al. Anti-signal recognition particle autoantibodies: marker of a necrotising myopathy. Ann Rheum Dis 2006;65(12):1635–8.

97. Christopher-Stine L, Casciola-Rosen LA, Hong G, et al. A novel autoantibody recognizing 200-kd and 100-kd proteins is associated with an immune-mediated necrotizing myopathy. Arthritis Rheum 2010;62(9):2757–66.

98. Sarui H, Maruyama T, Ito I, et al. Necrotising myositis in Behcet's disease: characteristic features on magnetic resonance imaging and a review of the literature. Ann Rheum Dis 2002;61(8):751–2.

99. Sampson JB, Smith SM, Smith AG, et al. Paraneoplastic myopathy: response to intravenous immunoglobulin. Neuromuscul Disord 2007;17(5):404–8.

100. Levin N, Abramsky O, Lossos A, et al. Extrathymic malignancies in patients with myasthenia gravis. J Neurol Sci 2005;237(1/2):39–43.

101. Romi F, Skeie GO, Aarli JA, et al. Muscle autoantibodies in subgroups of myasthenia gravis patients. J Neurol 2000;247(5):369–75.

Metabolic Myopathies: Clinical Features and Diagnostic Approach

Edward C. Smith, MD[a], Areeg El-Gharbawy, MD[b],
Dwight D. Koeberl, MD, PhD[b],*

KEYWORDS

- Inherited disorders of metabolism • Metabolic myopathy
- Glycogen storage disease • Mitochondrial disorder
- Fatty acid oxidation

The metabolic myopathies are a heterogeneous group of disorders that share the common feature of inadequate production of cellular energy in the muscle (**Table 1**). These myopathies are often categorized as either hereditary (primary) disorders or acquired (secondary) disorders. A further clinical distinction can be made between those disorders associated with primarily dynamic features characterized by transient, exercise-induced fatigue, muscle cramping, and rhabdomyolysis and those disorders associated with primarily static features such as fixed weakness.

A detailed review of muscle energy metabolism is beyond the scope of this review, but a brief consideration of the pertinent metabolic pathways is useful to understand better this group of disorders. Under normal circumstances, energy for skeletal muscle function in the form adenosine triphosphate (ATP) is derived from muscle glycogen, blood glucose, and free fatty acids.[1] Each of these primary energy sources is metabolized through specific biochemical pathways into the final common product, ATP. The majority of fuel for muscle is provided by carbohydrates in the form of glycogen and by lipids in the form of free fatty acids. Through the process of anaerobic glycolysis, glycogen is metabolized to pyruvate inside the muscle cells (**Fig. 1**). Pyruvate is then decarboxylated into acetyl-coenzyme A (acetyl-CoA) inside the mitochondria. Similarly, β-oxidation of free fatty acids (fatty acid oxidation; FAO) inside mitochondria provides another source of acetyl-CoA (**Fig. 2**). Acetyl-CoA then enters

---

[a] Division of Pediatric Neurology, Department of Pediatrics, Duke University Medical Center, DUMC Box 3936, Durham, NC 27710, USA
[b] Division of Medical Genetics, Department of Pediatrics, Duke University Medical Center, DUMC Box 103856, Durham, NC 27710, USA
* Corresponding author.
E-mail address: dwight.koeberl@duke.edu

Rheum Dis Clin N Am 37 (2011) 201–217
doi:10.1016/j.rdc.2011.01.004
0889-857X/11/$ – see front matter © 2011 Elsevier Inc. All rights reserved.

Table 1
Classification of the metabolic myopathies

Disorder	Presentation	Provocation	Screening Laboratory Testing	Confirmatory Testing	Treatment	Differential Diagnosis	Inheritance	OMIM Number
Dynamic Myopathies								
McArdle disease (GSD V)	Acute rhabdomyolysis, second wind phenomenon	Vigorous exercise	Abnormal ischemic forearm test, ± elevated CK, elevated muscle glycogen content	Myophosphorylase gene mutation; phosphorylase activity	Oral sucrose before exercise	PK deficiency	Autosomal recessive	#232600
Carnitine palmitoyl transferase II (CPT II) deficiency	Delayed rhabdomyolysis	Fasting, prolonged exercise	Abnormal acylcarnitine profile when stressed, normal CK	CPT II gene mutation, CPT activity in fibroblasts or muscle	Carbohydrate ± MCT oil before exercise, avoidance of fasting	Disorders of β-oxidation of long-chain fatty acids	Autosomal recessive	#255110
Phosphofructokinase (PFK) deficiency (GSD VII/Tarui)	Exercise intolerance, muscle pain	Stressful illness, exercise	± Elevated CK, elevated muscle glycogen content	PFK gene mutation, PFK activity in muscle	High protein diet, aerobic conditioning	Mitochondrial disorders	Autosomal recessive	#232800
Phosphorylase b kinase (PK) deficiency (GSD IXd)[16]	Acute rhabdomyolysis	Vigorous exercise	± Elevated CK, elevated muscle glycogen content	PK gene mutation, PK activity in muscle	High protein diet	McArdle disease	Autosomal recessive or X-linked recessive	#300559
Static Myopathies								
Mitochondrial disorders (mitochondrial oxidative phosphorylation defects)	Exercise intolerance	Stressful illness, exercise	Abnormal urine organic acids, normal CK	Electron transport chain (ETC) testing in muscle, coenzyme Q_{10} in muscle	Coenzyme Q_{10}/ creatine monohydrate/α-lipoic acid supplementation	PFK deficiency	Autosomal recessive or maternal inheritance (mitochondrial DNA mutations)	MERRF #545000; Kearns-Sayre syndrome #530000; many others
Acid maltase deficiency (GSD II)/ Pompe disease	Proximal weakness	Not applicable	Elevated urinary glucose tetrasaccharide, baseline elevated CK, elevated muscle glycogen content	Acid α-glucosidase (GAA) gene mutations, GAA activity in blood, fibroblasts, muscle	Enzyme replacement with recombinant human GAA	Limb girdle muscular dystrophies	Autosomal recessive	#232300

Abbreviations: MCT, medium-chain triglyceride; MERRF, myoclonic epilepsy and ragged-red fibers; OMIM, Online Mendelian Inheritance in Man.

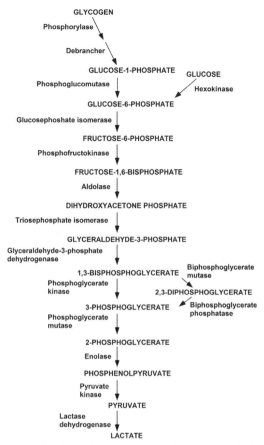

Fig. 1. Glycogenolytic and glycolytic enzymes involved in metabolic myopathies. The substrates and enzymes for each step are listed.

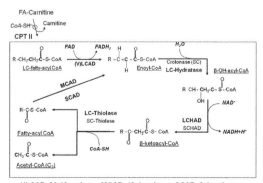

VLCAD: 20-12 carbons; MCAD: 12-4 carbons; SCAD: 6-4 carbons

Fig. 2. Fatty acid oxidation (FAO) spiral. Pathways in the FAO spiral are shown inside the box. The chain length specificity for the dehydrogenase enzymes is listed. CoA, coenzyme A; LCHAD, long-chain acyl-CoA dehydrogenase; MCAD, medium-chain acyl-CoA dehydrogenase; SC(H)AD, short-chain acyl-CoA dehydrogenase; VLCAD, very long-chain acyl-CoA dehydrogenase.

the Krebs cycle, generating reduced electron carriers that deliver electrons to the mitochondrial electron transport chain, thus driving the production of energy in the form of ATP (see **Fig. 1**). Defects in any one of the steps involved in this complex metabolic pathway can lead to an insufficient supply of ATP and an inability to sustain normal muscle function in times of increased metabolic demand.

The complex nature of the various metabolic pathways involved is reflected in the broad phenotypic presentation of many of these disorders (see **Table 1**). Classic symptoms of the metabolic myopathies, including early exertional fatigue, myalgias, muscle cramps or contractures, and myoglobinuria, may emerge during times of high energy demand due to exercise, illness, or fasting. Because the predominant energy substrate varies as a function of the intensity and duration of exercise, a detailed clinical history can often provide important diagnostic clues. Glycogen breakdown provides substrates for cellular energy production during rapid, vigorous exercise, whereas FAO acts as the main player during prolonged exercise and/or fasting. At rest, free fatty acids provide the major energy source for skeletal muscle via aerobic metabolism. By contrast, brief, high-intensity (isometric) exercise such as weight-lifting relies heavily on anaerobic glycogenolysis for a rapid, short-lived energy supply. The primary source of energy for muscle for light-to-moderate intensity exercise of short duration is predominantly glucose and free fatty acids. As exercise duration increases glycogen stores are depleted, and the demand for free fatty acid–derived energy increases. This process explains the characteristic pattern of muscle fatigue, stiffness, cramping, and myalgias that occur shortly after brief, maximal exertion in the myogenic forms of glycogen storage diseases (GSDs). By contrast, symptoms associated with disorders of lipid metabolism typically appear after prolonged, moderate-intensity exercise, such as jogging or swimming. Thus, patients with McArdle disease (GSD type V) become symptomatic during intense exercise, whereas in carnitine palmitoyltransferase II (CPT II) deficiency, an FAO disorder, patients present following sustained exercise and other metabolic stressors (see **Table 1**).

The variable and often transient nature of these symptoms can present a challenging diagnostic dilemma. Depending on the underlying metabolic defect, some patients may present in infancy or early childhood, whereas others may not present until well into adulthood. Furthermore, some disorders may be strictly limited to muscle pathology whereas others, particularly those involving mitochondrial dysfunction, may demonstrate multisystem involvement. To make a proper diagnosis, it also becomes necessary to recognize other inherited and acquired conditions mimicking metabolic myopathies.

Several acquired and inherited conditions may mimic metabolic myopathies, and must be properly diagnosed both to avoid unnecessary and potentially harmful therapies and to allow appropriate treatment and counseling (**Box 1**). For example, statins, a common group of drugs used for treatment of hypercholesterolemia, has emerged as a cause of iatrogenic myalgia.[2] The precise mechanism of muscle injury in statin-induced myopathy is unknown, but there appears to be a dose-related effect, with higher doses leading to myopathy and rhabdomyolysis. A recent study has shown an increased risk for statin-induced myopathy in patients harboring a common single-nucleotide polymorphism in the *SLCO1B1* gene on chromosome 12. This gene is involved in the hepatic uptake of statin drugs.[3] The incidence of homozygosity or heterozygosity for mutations associated with rare metabolic myopathies was increased in a large group of patients evaluated for statin-induced myopathy. Muscle coenzyme Q_{10} deficiency was highly prevalent in this group,[4] and their response to supplementation remains to be established; however, this biochemical abnormality could shed light on the pathogenesis of statin-induced myopathy.

Box 1
Causes of myalgia other than metabolic myopathies

1. Inflammatory myopathy (dermatomyositis, polymyositis, inclusion body myositis)

2. Necrotizing, noninflammatory myopathies (paraneoplastic, anti–signal recognition particle)

3. Infection (viral)

4. Toxin/drug-induced (ethanol, statins, cyclosporine, colchicine)

5. Endocrinopathies (hypo-/hyperthyroidism, hypo-/hyperparathyroidism, diabetes mellitus)

6. Polymyalgia rheumatica

7. Fibromyalgia

8. Benign cramp-fasciculation syndrome

9. Restless leg syndrome

10. Muscular dystrophies (dystrophinopathies, limb girdle muscular dystrophy)

11. Myotonic disorders (myotonic dystrophy type 2, myotonia congenita)

12. Motor neuron disease (amyotrophic lateral sclerosis, spinal muscular atrophy)

Other myopathies that may mimic metabolic myopathies include limb-girdle muscular dystrophies or, more commonly, chronic inflammatory myopathies such as polymyositis. Systemic manifestations such as a rash, malaise, interstitial fibrosis, carditis, and gastrointestinal dysfunction may suggest the presence of an acquired inflammatory myopathy, but the distinction can be difficult. For a more detailed discussion, the reader is referred to an excellent review of the subject.[1]

Many tools are available to the clinician to aid in the diagnostic evaluation of metabolic myopathies. As discussed later with each group of disorders, one of the most cost-effective and least invasive tools remains the clinical history and physical examination that can provide invaluable information, allowing the clinician to narrow or broaden further diagnostic testing as appropriate and avoid unnecessary invasive testing. A thorough history and examination will often help differentiate a dynamic myopathy characterized by transient, severe symptoms from a static myopathy characterized by fixed weakness (see **Table 1**). As the primary metabolic myopathies are hereditary, a thorough, targeted family history may provide valuable information. Once a thorough history and physical examination have been performed, routine laboratory tests including serum electrolytes, glucose, liver transaminases, creatine kinase (CK), lactate, ammonia, and urinalysis may be useful. In some cases, electromyography (EMG) and routine muscle biopsy may provide valuable information (see **Table 1; Table 2**), but they are often normal. The forearm ischemic exercise test has been reviewed elsewhere and may be helpful as well, particularly if GSD type V is suspected.[1] Further diagnostic tests such as urine organic acids, plasma amino acids, and plasma acylcarnitine profile may provide more specific results, allowing the clinician to approach more costly confirmatory testing, including enzyme and/or DNA analysis on leukocytes, fibroblasts, and/or liver, in a rational, potentially cost-effective manner (see **Table 2**).

Metabolic myopathies are broadly grouped into 3 categories based on the underlying metabolic defect: (1) muscle glycogenoses, (2) disorders of FAO, and (3) mitochondrial myopathies. The following discussion focuses on the most common primary metabolic myopathies associated with primarily dynamic symptoms characterized by exercise-induced myalgia, early fatigue, cramping, and myoglobinuria.

Table 2
Diagnostic testing in metabolic myopathies

Disorder	Blood, Urine (u)	Cultured Fibroblasts	Muscle Histology	Muscle Enzymology[a]
GSDs				
GSD II	GAA, Hex$_4$ (u)	GAA	PAS	GAA, glycogen content
GSD V	Mutation screen, gene sequencing	N.A.	PAS	Myophosphorylase, glycogen content
GSD VII	Gene sequencing	N.A.	PAS (occasionally revealing)	PFK, glycogen content (occasionally elevated)
GSD IX	Gene sequencing (4 genes), phosphorylase kinase (XL only)	N.A.	PAS	PK, glycogen content
Other GSD	Gene sequencing, if available	N.A.	PAS (occasionally revealing)	Specific enzyme assays, glycogen content (occasionally elevated)
FATMO Disorders				
CPT II deficiency	Plasma acylcarnitine profile (when symptomatic), mutation screen (limited sensitivity), gene sequencing	CPT II	Lipid myopathy (?)	CPT II

LCHAD/Tri-functional protein, VLCAD, or MAD deficiency	Plasma acylcarnitine profile, mutation screen (limited sensitivity), gene sequencing, urine organic acids (MAD deficiency)	Enzyme assay, in vitro probe (limited sensitivity)	Lipid myopathy (?)	Specific enzyme assays (not usually needed, given less invasive testing)
Mitochondrial Disorders				
Respiratory chain defects	Gene sequencing (targeted, limited sensitivity), organic acids (u), plasma lactate (limited sensitivity)	ETC (limited sensitivity)	Ragged red fibers or cytochrome c oxidase deficiency (limited sensitivity)	Respiratory chain/ETC (freshly isolated mitochondria preferred, limited availability)
Coenzyme Q$_{10}$ deficiency	Gene sequencing (limited sensitivity)	ETC (limited sensitivity)		Coenzyme Q$_{10}$, respiratory chain/ETC (freshly isolated mitochondria preferred, limited availability)

Abbreviations: CPT II, carnitine palmitoyltransferase II; ETC, electron transport chain testing; FATMO, fatty acid transport and mitochondrial oxidation; GAA, acid α-glucosidase; GSD, glycogen storage disease; LCHAD, long-chain acyl-CoA dehydrogenase; MAD, multiple acyl-CoA dehydrogenase; N.A., not available; PAS, periodic acid-Schiff; PFK, phosphofructokinase; PK, phosphorylase *b* kinase; VLCAD, very long-chain acyl-CoA dehydrogenase.
^a Requires flash-frozen sample, 50–1000 mg.

DISORDERS OF GLYCOGEN METABOLISM (MUSCLE GLYCOGENOSES)

The classification of GSDs is based on the associated enzyme defect and clinical presentation. Two GSDs do not involve skeletal muscle: GSD type I (von Gierke disease) and GSD type VI (Hers disease).[3] Some GSDs produce primarily static symptoms of fixed, proximal weakness, including GSD type II (Pompe disease), GSD type III (Cori-Forbes disease), and GSD type IV (Andersen disease). The latter 2 disorders are typified primarily by liver involvement and are not further discussed here. Late-onset Pompe disease causes progressive, proximal muscle weakness that may progress to respiratory failure, and it falls into the static myopathy category (see **Table 1**). Phosphofructokinase deficiency (GSD type VII; PFK deficiency, or Tarui disease) might be underdiagnosed, because it presents with nonspecific exercise intolerance and myalgias. Until recently, Tarui disease could only be diagnosed by functional enzyme testing requiring muscle biopsy. The diagnostic evaluation has been simplified with the recent availability of gene testing. The remaining disorders are rare, with the exception of McArdle disease (GSD type V), and typically produce dynamic symptoms.

GSD Type V (McArdle Disease)

GSD type V (Mendelian Inheritance in Man [MIM] #232600) is caused by homozygous or compound heterozygous mutations in the *PYGM* gene, which encodes the skeletal muscle isoform of glycogen phosphorylase, also known as myophosphorylase, an essential enzyme for glycogenolysis. As the heart and liver isoforms are not affected, the disease exclusively affects skeletal muscle.[2] The typical age of onset is in late childhood. Patients develop exercise intolerance, myalgia, and stiffness or weakness during brief, isometric exercise such as weight lifting or during prolonged moderate-intensity exercise such as jogging or swimming. Strenuous exercise results in painful cramps and muscle swelling in those muscles that are actively engaged, which may last for hours. Myoglobinuria is seen in about 50% of the patients. Improvement in symptoms after a brief rest, the so-called second-wind phenomenon, is frequently reported. Approximately 50% of patients develop fixed weakness and muscle atrophy with aging.[4]

Serum CK levels are usually elevated at baseline in McArdle disease, and myogenic hyperuricemia results from excessive increase of adenosine diphosphate during exercise. EMG is typically normal. The forearm exercise test will demonstrate a normal increase in ammonia levels without an increase in lactate or pyruvate levels. A similar pattern is seen in the other muscle GSDs with the exception of Pompe disease, brancher enzyme deficiency (GSD type IV), and phosphorylase *b* kinase deficiency (GSD type IX). Muscle biopsy will demonstrate absent or severely reduced myophosphorylase staining on histochemical analysis. Enzyme analysis of flash-frozen muscle can confirm the diagnosis by demonstrating absent or reduced myophosphorylase activity. Current molecular genetic testing on blood can detect mutations that account for about 90% of cases, avoiding the need for biopsy.[2]

In the absence of well-established treatment of McArdle disease, several therapeutic interventions have been proposed. Supplementation with creatine monohydrate, branched-chain amino acids, or pyridoxine (vitamin B6) were reported as beneficial, although results have been variable. A diet rich in complex carbohydrates combined with regular aerobic exercise is advocated by many investigators. Recently, it has been clearly shown that consumption of approximately 40 g of sucrose or fructose shortly before vigorous physical exercise dramatically reduces symptoms.[5] Intense isometric exercise limited to isolated muscle groups should be avoided.

GSD Type VII (Tarui Disease)

Phosphofructokinase (PFK) deficiency (MIM #232800) is a well-characterized glycolysis defect with primarily muscle involvement. PFK is a rate-limiting enzyme, acting at the third step of glycolysis where it catalyzes the phosphorylation of fructose-6-phosphate to fructose-1,6-bisphosphate. A defect in PFK results in a block in muscle glycolysis and glycogenolysis, thus limiting ATP regeneration from glycolysis, and impairing oxidative phosphorylation and energy production.[6] PFK is composed of 3 subunits expressed in a tissue-specific manner: muscle (M), liver (L), and platelet (P). Deficiency of the M subunit results in myopathy, while partial loss of PFK activity in red blood cells (RBCs) leads to compensated hemolysis because the muscle type contributes to 50% of the total erythrocyte enzyme activity while the liver type contributes the other half.[6] Four clinical forms of PFK deficiency have been characterized.[7] The classic form (GSD type VIIa) includes exercise intolerance, muscle cramps, muscle pain, and myoglobinuria after exercise. Patients with the late-onset form (GSD type VIIb) usually do not show any apparent myopathy during childhood, but may experience exercise intolerance starting in childhood. Slowly progressive weakness becomes apparent in the fifth decade and can lead to significant disability. The infantile form (GSD type VIIc) presents soon after birth. Infants are severely hypotonic and usually die within the first year of life. The molecular basis of GSD type VIIc has not been confirmed (Salvatore Dimauro, Columbia University, personal communication, 2009). The fourth form is characterized by hereditary, nonspherocytic hemolytic anemia without muscle symptoms, thus distinguishing it from the other forms of GSD VII.[7]

An "out-of-wind" phenomenon has been observed in patients with Tarui disease, which correlated with increased glucose production and, presumably, decreased availability of free fatty acids and ketones for ATP production.[8] This feature distinguishes GSD type VII from McArdle disease (GSD type V) in which patients develop a second-wind phenomenon as a result of a metabolic block restricted to glycogenolysis.[8] Other distinguishing features of GSD type V may include mild reticulocytosis and increased serum bilirubin.

Enzymatic activity of PFK in muscle is usually completely lost, with no clear evidence of a relationship between the residual PFK enzyme activity in skeletal muscle and phenotype expression of the disease. Normally structured glycogen accumulates in the muscle of some patients with GSD type VII. Alternatively, an abnormal polysaccharide (polyglucosan) is found in muscle fibers in addition to excess glycogen in a few patients. The abnormal polysaccharide stains with periodic acid-Schiff and is more often found in GSD VIIb [7] The muscle in PFK deficiency may show vacuolar formation in the subsarcolemmal space.[9] Two mutations comprise the great majority of Tarui disease alleles among Ashkenazi Jewish patients, $\Delta 5$ and ΔC-22.[10] At present there is no specific form of treatment, and treatment is symptomatic, including the avoidance of strenuous exercise and aggressive treatment of myoglobinuria.[11] However, one patient with infantile PFK deficiency and arthrogryposis responded favorably to a ketogenic diet, suggesting that a high fat content diet may be beneficial in patients with PFK deficiency.[12]

Phosphoglycerate Kinase Deficiency

Phosphoglycerate kinase (PGK) deficiency (MIM #300653), is a multisystem disorder involving the RBC, the central nervous system (CNS), and muscle. PGK deficiency is the only X-linked disorder of glycolysis.[13] PGK acts in the terminal glycolytic pathway yielding 3-phosphoglycerate and ATP (see **Fig. 1**). Manifesting females present with anemia, whereas hemizygous males have additional features suggestive of CNS and/or muscle disease. CNS manifestations may include behavioral abnormalities, emotional lability, mental retardation, epilepsy, movement disorders, or hemiplegia and aphasia. A 4-base deletion in exon 6 of the *PGK* gene caused isolated exertional myopathy and myoglobinuria in an adult male.[14] As in other glycolytic disorders, the specific diagnosis is made by measuring PGK activity in muscle and erythrocytes. CK elevation occurs during the forearm ischemic exercise test, which reveals normal blood pyruvate and lactate increase in patients with the muscle phenotype. Although there is no specific treatment, a ketogenic diet was postulated to be beneficial, as it would theoretically bypass the defect in glycolysis.[15]

GSD Type IXd

Phosphorylase *b* kinase (PHK) deficiency is a rare GSD (GSD type IXd; MIM #300559).[3] It is considered a mild metabolic myopathy characterized by impaired lactate production during moderate-intensity dynamic exercise, mild elevations of plasma CK and muscle glycogen content, and a possible improvement of exercise tolerance with intravenous glucose infusion.[16] Only the muscle-specific α-subunit (PHKA1) is X-linked. Deficiency of PHK, the activating enzyme of muscle phosphorylase, is thought to cause similar effects on muscle glycogenolysis as in McArdle disease, albeit with the retention of residual myophosphorylase activity. Accordingly, the clinical features of PHK deficiency can mimic those of McArdle disease but are less pronounced. Residual PHK activity is observed in all patients and is possibly caused by the β-subunit of the enzyme, which has the capacity to phosphorylate myophosphorylase and is inherited in an autosomal recessive manner.

GSD Type X

Phosphoglycerate mutase (PGAM) deficiency (GSD type X; MIM #261670), has been considered a relatively benign muscle glycogenosis.[17] PGAM is an enzyme of terminal glycolysis that catalyzes the reversible shift of the phosphate group between C-2 and C-3 of glycerate (see **Fig. 1**). The prevalence of the disease appears to be more common in African Americans; however, cases have been reported in patients from Italy, Japan, and of Pakistani descent. A nonsense mutation (W78X) in exon 1 of the *PGAM2* gene encoding the muscle subunit has been commonly found in African American patients, suggesting a founder effect in this population.[17] Patients are asymptomatic until they perform brief strenuous exercise, which triggers myalgias, muscle cramps, and often muscle necrosis and myoglobinuria. The benign clinical phenotype has been attributed to residual PGAM activity, which was thought to be sufficient to allow near normal oxidative capacity and production of lactate during exercise.[18] CK may be elevated, and forearm ischemic exercise testing shows mildly increased venous lactate.[19] Muscle biopsy shows normal to mild glycogen accumulation, with prominent tubular aggregates.

GSD Type XIII

β-Enolase deficiency (GSD XIII; MIM #612932) is a muscle-specific enolase deficiency known as glycogenosis type XIII. The enzyme catalyzes the conversion of 2-phospho-D-glycerate to 2-phospho-enolpyruvate, one of the terminal steps of glycolysis (see **Fig. 1**). Patients with β-enolase deficiency present with exercise-induced myalgias, and increased CK levels after intense exercise. Symptoms may be episodic for years, with no lactate increase induced by ischemic exercise. The muscle biopsy does not show gross glycogen accumulation, although an increased amount of sarcoplasmic glycogen β particles may be detected by electron microscopy.[20] A distinguishing feature from other glycolytic defects, such as PFK and PGK deficiencies, is the lack of nonmuscular tissue involvement attributable to muscle-specific expression of the *ENO3* gene.[20]

Lactate Dehydrogenase Deficiency

Lactate dehydrogenase (LDH) deficiency (GSD XI; MIM #612933) is a rare disorder of glycolysis associated with metabolic myopathy.[21] LDH plays a role in the final steps of glycolysis by catalyzing the conversion of pyruvate to lactate with nicotinamide adenine dinucleotide as a cofactor (see **Fig. 1**). Clinical features are related to diminished energy supply and impaired ability to sustain exercise due to muscle pain and stiffness. Patients present with intolerance to intense exercise, cramps, and recurrent myoglobinuria, all of variable severity. A distinctive feature of LDH deficiency is the high level of CK contrasted with low levels of serum LDH during episodes of myglobinuria.

Phosphoglucomutase Deficiency

Phosphoglucomutase (PGM1) deficiency (GSD type XIV; MIM #612934) has been recently described in a patient who presented with exercise intolerance and episodic rhabdomyolysis.[22] The patient had a normal elevation of lactate and ammonia on forearm-exercise test. In vitro analysis of muscle anaerobic glycogenolysis and glycolysis revealed a metabolic block after the formation of glucose-1-phosphate and before formation of glucose-6-phosphate, indicating PGM1 deficiency (see **Fig. 1**). Muscle histopathology revealed abnormal subsarcolemmal and sarcoplasmic accumulations of normally structured, free glycogen. Biochemical investigation of muscle revealed a marked reduction of PGM1 activity whereas muscle phosphorylase and PFK activities were normal. *PGM1* gene sequencing revealed de novo compound heterozygous mutations.[22]

Fatty Acid Oxidation Disorders

FAO (β-oxidation of fatty acids) is the major source of energy during periods of sustained, low-intensity exercise or prolonged fasting. In infants, these disorders typically present during periods of illness or poor oral intake. In children and adults, exercise intolerance and myoglobinuria are the most common presenting features. The major disorders of lipid metabolism that present with isolated myopathy include: (1) carnitine palmitoyltransferase II (CPT II) deficiency, (2) very long-chain acyl-CoA dehydrogenase (VLCAD) deficiency, and (3) long-chain acyl-CoA dehydrogenase (LCHAD) or trifunctional protein (TFP).[23] Of these, CPT II deficiency is the most prevalent and is the most common overall cause of hereditary, recurrent myoglobinuria.

CPT II deficiency

CPT II deficiency (MIM #255110) can be classified into 3 different presentations: (1) a lethal neonatal form involving multiorgan failure, (2) a severe infantile hepatocardiomuscular form, and (3) a milder, purely myopathic form. The severity of disease appears to be related to the type of mutation. Missense mutations that allow production of some partially functional enzyme activity are typically found in the milder myopathic form, whereas protein-truncating mutations produce the more severe neonatal and infantile phenotypes.[10]

CPT II is a protein located on the inner surface of the inner mitochondrial membrane, and serves a critical role in the conversion of long-chain acylcarnitines back into long-chain acyl-CoA species (see **Fig. 2**). Long-chain acyl-CoA species subsequently undergo β-oxidation, which provides acetyl-CoA to the tricarboxylic acid cycle and drives synthesis of ATP via the electron transport chain. The sequential reduction in acyl-CoA chain length through 4 sequential enzymatic steps has been termed the "FAO spiral" (see **Fig. 2**).

In contrast to the muscle glycogenoses, the myopathic form of CPT II deficiency often does not produce cramps, and muscle weakness should not be present between attacks. Serum CK levels are usually normal, as are EMG and muscle pathology. Patients may complain of muscle weakness and myalgia triggered by exercise, infection, or fasting. Other triggers include cold exposure and general anesthesia. Age of onset is typically in childhood but can vary widely. The plasma acylcarnitine profile, showing elevated C16, C18:1, and C18:2, serves as a screening test that will most often detect CPT II deficiency when the patient is symptomatic; however, functional enzyme analysis of fibroblasts or muscle tissue presumably offers higher sensitivity.[23] Diagnosis can be confirmed by whole blood DNA analysis that will detect known mutations in roughly 80% of patients.[24]

Patients with CPT II deficiency are instructed to avoid prolonged fasting (>10 hours). Sustained, intensive exercise should be avoided, and carbohydrate loading before and during exercise may prevent attacks. Dietary supplementation with medium-chain triglycerides provides an alternative substrate for FAO involving long-chain fatty acids.[25]

FAO disorders involving long-chain acyl-CoA intermediates

VLCAD deficiency (MIM #201475) involves the first step in the FAO of long-chain acyl-CoA intermediates of 20 to 12 carbons in length (see **Fig. 2**), and as such affects tissues dependent on FAO for cellular energy production including liver, heart, and skeletal muscle. Clinical manifestations vary from lethal, infantile presentations with dilated cardiomyopathy and hypoketotic hypoglycemia to milder, later-onset myopathic presentations.[23] Typically the acylcarnitine profile from plasma or a blood-spot sample demonstrates elevated C14, C14:1, and C14:2 species, consistent with a block in oxidation of long-chain acyl-CoA species. Patients with VLCAD deficiency have a high risk for recurrent rhabdomyolysis associated with exercise or intercurrent illness, although treatment with a diet restricted in long-chain fats accompanied by medium-chain triglyceride supplementation provides generally effective treatment for this and other long-chain FAO defects described here.

More recently, VLCAD deficiency and other FAO defects involving long-chain species have been detected by expanded newborn screening.[26,27] The newborn screening experience with VLCAD deficiency emphasized the need for mutation and enzyme testing to confirm VLCAD deficiency whenever C14:1 is elevated in the initial newborn screening sample, as the C14:1 level may normalize following the neonatal period in the well-compensated, stable infant with VLCAD deficiency.[26]

Isolated LCHAD deficiency (MIM #609016) is a defect of one function from TFP (MIM #609015). Both LCHAD and complete TFP deficiency present similarly with elevated hydroxyl long-chain acylcarnitines (OH-C16, OH-C18:1, and OH-C18:2) in the acylcarnitine profile. LCHAD deficiency features long-term complications caused by cardiomyopathy, neuropathy, and retinopathy, with a high risk for rhabdomyolysis associated with stress or exercise.[27] TFP deficiency is more severe, with a high risk for early mortality.[27] Enzyme and mutation testing will differentiate isolated LCHAD deficiency from TFP deficiency. Moreover, the high prevalence of a common mutation in LCHAD deficiency, c.1528G>C, facilitates diagnosis. A unique feature of these disorders is the high frequency of third-trimester complications when the fetus is affected with LCHAD or TFP deficiency, including HELLP (Hemolysis, Elevated Liver enzymes, Low Platelets) and acute fatty liver of pregnancy, attributed to increased needs for ketogenesis in the maternal liver.[23] Treatment is as already described for

VLCAD deficiency, with additional care to prevent essential fatty acid deficiencies that might be associated with increased risk of retinopathy in LCHAD deficiency.[23,28]

Mitochondrial Oxidative Phosphorylation Disorders

Defects of mitochondrial oxidative phosphorylation are typified by multisystem involvement frequently involving muscle.[1] Not infrequently, though, mitochondrial disorders manifest as isolated myopathies in adults, as opposed to the encephalopathy and multisystem involvement associated with more classic infantile presentations. Late-onset mitochondrial myopathies feature proximal muscle weakness, easy fatigability, and variably elevated CK levels (see **Table 1**). Lactic acidemia is often absent. Thus, mitochondrial myopathies are frequently misdiagnosed as inflammatory myopathy on presentation.

Classification by the underlying gene defect is complicated by tremendous genetic heterogeneity, with approximately 20% of mutations involving mitochondrial DNA and the remainder affecting numerous nuclear genes. Using the modified Walker criteria is essential to confirming the diagnosis of a mitochondrial myopathy, because the presence of both characteristic clinical symptoms and diagnostic laboratory testing are required for confirmation of affected status.[29] Muscle histology may feature ragged-red fibers (**Fig. 3**) and decreased cytochrome c oxidase (COX) staining, or it may be normal. Functional enzymology on flash-frozen muscle tissue or fibroblasts allows quantitative assessment of electron transport chain (ETC) complex activities. In

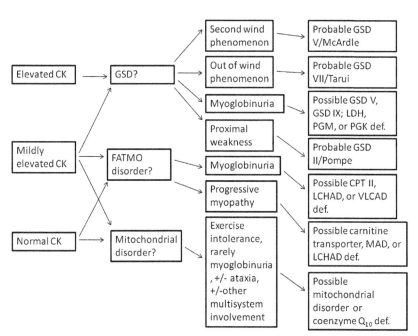

Fig. 3. Diagnostic flowchart. Schematic for the investigation of likely causes for metabolic myopathies, given presence or absence of creatine kinase elevations. CK, creatine kinase; def., deficiency; CPT II, carnitine palmitoyltransferase II; FATMO, fatty acid transport and mitochondrial oxidation; GSD, glycogen storage disease; LCHAD, long-chain acyl-CoA dehydrogenase; LDH, lactate dehydrogenase; MAD, multiple acyl-CoA dehydrogenase; PGK, phosphoglycerate kinase; PGM, phosphoglucomutase; VLCAD, very long-chain acyl-CoA dehydrogenase.

general, the mitochondrial myopathies are most effectively diagnosed via studies on flash-frozen muscle tissue, which will demonstrate abnormalities on ETC enzymology testing. Flash-frozen muscle samples offer greater sensitivity than skin fibroblasts, but special handling required to maintain sample integrity is cumbersome, and frequently delays or prevents the diagnosis. Noninvasive testing can be useful in some cases, either through ETC testing of cultured fibroblasts or mutation testing of a blood sample (see **Table 2** and **Fig. 1**).

Mitochondrial myopathies are emerging as a more frequent cause of metabolic myopathy than previously recognized. However, multisystem involvement is more typical for mitochondrial cytopathies, and this fact can help contrast these disorders from the aforementioned GSDs (reviewed previously[30]). Neurologic manifestations are common in patients with mitochondrial disorders, including seizures, strokes, ophthalmoplegia, retinopathy, ataxia, sensorineural hearing loss, peripheral neuropathy, and myopathy. Classically the mitochondrial myopathies were associated with point mutations in mitochondrial tRNA genes (eg, myoclonic epilepsy and ragged-red fibers [MERRF]; MIM #545000) or large deletions involving the mitochondrial genome (eg, Kearns-Sayre syndrome; MIM #530000).[31] MERRF features myoclonic epilepsy, ataxia, and myopathy, and muscle histochemistry reveals ragged fibers. Family history may reveal maternal inheritance of features such as cervical lipomas and cardiovascular disease, which are associated with a causative point mutation at position 8344 in the mitochondrial genome involving the tRNA for leucine. Only maternal relatives are at risk, because mitochondria are inherited almost exclusively through cytoplasmic inheritance in the oocytes. The position 8344 mutation conveniently can be detected by mutation testing of blood samples. However, MERRF comprises only a small subset of the mitochondrial myopathies and, therefore, muscle biopsy testing is a more reliable method for detection of these disorders. Kearns-Sayre syndrome is characterized by the triad of ptosis, pigmentary retinopathy, and cardiac conduction defects, and the underlying deletion of mitochondrial DNA almost always arises as a sporadic mutation.

Occasionally mitochondrial myopathies have been associated with point mutations in the mitochondrial genome, discovered through muscle testing in association the deficiency of one or more ETC complexes. Alternatively, isolated myopathy has been reported more frequently in mitochondrial disorders caused by the depletion of mitochondrial genomic DNA or coenzyme Q_{10} synthesis defects, detailed below.

An alternative cause of mitochondrial disorders is nuclear gene defects that interfere with mitochondrial (mt) DNA replication, thereby causing mtDNA depletion. Three general presentations have been recognized in association with mtDNA depletion: isolated myopathy, encephalomyopathy, or hepatocerebral syndrome.[32] Isolated myopathy has been linked with *thymidine kinase (TK) 2* gene mutations inherited in an autosomal recessive manner. Whereas initial symptoms occur in infancy, consisting of failure to thrive, hypotonia, and muscle weakness accompanied by elevated CK, the clinical course progresses to death from pulmonary insufficiency in the first to second decade. Muscle histochemistry reveals decreased COX staining and gradual appearance of ragged-red fibers. Quantitative mtDNA analysis reveals mtDNA depletion. *TK2* mutations have been demonstrated in approximately 20% of myopathic mtDNA depletion syndrome.

More recently, the deficiency of coenzyme Q_{10} synthesis has emerged as a cause for isolated mitochondrial myopathy.[2] Coenzyme Q_{10} synthesis defects have been implicated in several presentations, including encephalomyopathy with recurrent myoglobinuria and ragged-red fibers; encephalopathy, lactic acidemia, and nephropathy; cerebellar ataxia with oculomotor apraxia and hypogonadotropic hypogonadism; Leigh syndrome with growth retardation, ataxia, and deafness; and adult-onset myopathy with exercise intolerance, proximal weakness, and elevated CK and lactate. Establishing the diagnosis of coenzyme Q_{10} deficiency requires quantification of coenzyme Q_{10} in flash-frozen muscle (see **Table 2**).

Of note, the underlying gene defect in cases of isolated myopathy has involved the electron transferring protein dehydrogenase (*ETFDH*) gene that was previously described in patients with multiple acyl-CoA dehydrogenase (MAD) deficiency (glutaric acidemia type II; MIM #231680).[33] Previous reports attributed MAD deficiency to a "trifunctional protein deficiency,"[1] creating confusion with a well-recognized TFP that affects 3 enzyme functions in FAO including LCHAD (see earlier discussion).[23]

Treatment of mitochondrial disorders involves supplementation with coenzyme Q_{10} and other cofactors that increase oxidative phosphorylation. Coenzyme $Q_{10,}$ in combination with creatine monohydrate and α-lipoic acid was beneficial in one series.[34] Diagnosing coenzyme Q_{10} deficiency myopathy provides the great benefit of confirming the value of high-dose coenzyme Q_{10} supplementation.

SUMMARY: APPROACH TO THE DIAGNOSIS OF METABOLIC MYOPATHIES

Firmly establishing a diagnosis of a metabolic myopathy is critical for several reasons, including the potential for therapeutic intervention and a need to provide the patient with prognostic information and appropriate genetic counseling. Proper diagnosis also avoids unnecessary testing and inappropriate therapies such as immunomodulatory therapy for a suspected acquired process. A carefully designed evaluation, guided by clinical and laboratory information (see **Fig. 1**), will allow proper diagnosis with minimally invasive testing.

When presented with a patient with recurrent rhabdomyolysis, muscle cramps, and a clear second-wind phenomenon, McArdle disease should be suspected and appropriate molecular genetic testing should be pursued. By contrast, exercise intolerance accompanied by weakness that is exacerbated by carbohydrate intake, the so-called out-of-wind phenomenon, suggests GSD type VII (PFK deficiency) that might be confirmed through gene sequencing or muscle enzyme testing if necessary (see **Fig. 1**). At times, reaching the diagnosis will require more invasive testing including histology, histochemistry, and enzyme analysis of muscle tissue, such as is commonly the case with the mitochondrial myopathies (see **Table 2**). Establishing the diagnosis of CPT II deficiency frequently requires enzyme testing of cultured fibroblasts or muscle, because mutation testing often identifies only a single mutation.

Progressing from careful clinical evaluation to the least invasive testing likely to yield a diagnosis, and finally to the muscle biopsy when necessary, is a reasonable strategy. Several biochemical genetics laboratories offer "myoglobinuria panels," which can facilitate enzyme testing. If the decision is made to proceed to muscle biopsy, the importance of careful planning to ensure adequate sampling, processing, and preservation cannot be overstated. Collaboration with all of the consultants involved, including the rheumatologist, metabolic specialist, neurologist, surgeon, primary physician, pathologist, and biochemical laboratory director under the direction of an identified team leader, will enhance the chances of establishing a correct diagnosis in a timely, cost-effective manner. The metabolic myopathies are a large, heterogeneous group of disorders with wide phenotypic variability, and thus remain diagnostically challenging. These disorders should remain in the differential diagnosis for any patient with muscle pain, fatigue, and recurrent rhabdomyolysis, particularly when associated with exercise. A stepwise, comprehensive diagnostic approach is necessary to maximize diagnostic yield and spare patients unnecessary therapies, interventions, and costs.

ACKNOWLEDGMENTS

We wish to thank our patients and colleagues for their support and understanding while we developed the concepts underlying this article. We thank Dr David Millington for the illustration of the FAO spiral.

REFERENCES

1. Wortmann RL, DiMauro S. Differentiating idiopathic inflammatory myopathies from metabolic myopathies. Rheum Dis Clin North Am 2002;28:759–78.
2. Quinzii CM, Hirano M, DiMauro S. CoQ10 deficiency diseases in adults. Mitochondrion 2007;7(Suppl):S122–6.
3. Chen YT. Glycogen storage diseases. In: Scriver CR, Beaudet AL, Sly WS, et al, editors, The metabolic and molecular bases of inherited disease, vol. 8. New York: McGraw-Hill; 2001. p. 1521–51.
4. DiMauro S, Lamperti C. Muscle glycogenoses. Muscle Nerve 2001;24:984–99.
5. Andersen ST, Haller RG, Vissing J. Effect of oral sucrose shortly before exercise on work capacity in McArdle disease. Arch Neurol 2008;65:786–9.
6. Tarui S. Glycolytic defects in muscle: aspects of collaboration between basic science and clinical medicine. Muscle Nerve 1995;3:S2–9.
7. Nakajima H, Raben N, Hamaguchi T, et al. Phosphofructokinase deficiency; past, present and future. Curr Mol Med 2002;2:197–212.
8. Vissing J, Galbo H, Haller RG. Paradoxically enhanced glucose production during exercise in humans with blocked glycolysis caused by muscle phosphofructokinase deficiency. Neurology 1996;47:766–71.
9. Agamanolis DP, Askari AD, Di Mauro S, et al. Muscle phosphofructokinase deficiency: two cases with unusual polysaccharide accumulation and immunologically active enzyme protein. Muscle Nerve 1980;3:456–67.
10. Sherman JB, Raben N, Nicastri C, et al. Common mutations in the phosphofructokinase-M gene in Ashkenazi Jewish patients with glycogenesis VII—and their population frequency. Am J Hum Genet 1994;55:305–13.
11. Heyne N, Guthoff M, Weisel KC. Rhabdomyolysis and acute kidney injury. N Engl J Med 2009;361:1412–3.
12. Swoboda KJ, Specht L, Jones HR, et al. Infantile phosphofructokinase deficiency with arthrogryposis: clinical benefit of a ketogenic diet. J Pediatr 1997;131:932–4.
13. Tsujino S, Shanske S, DiMauro S. Molecular genetic heterogeneity of phosphoglycerate kinase (PGK) deficiency. Muscle Nerve 1995;3:S45–9.
14. Hamano T, Mutoh T, Sugie H, et al. Phosphoglycerate kinase deficiency: an adult myopathic form with a novel mutation. Neurology 2000;54:1188–90.
15. De Vivo DC, Leary L, Wang D. Glucose transporter 1 deficiency syndrome and other glycolytic defects. J Child Neurol 2002;17(Suppl 3):3S15–3S23.
16. Ørngreen MC, Schelhaas HJ, Jeppesen TD, et al. Is muscle glycogenolysis impaired in X-linked phosphorylase b kinase deficiency? Neurology 2008;70: 1876–82.
17. Naini A, Toscano A, Musumeci O, et al. Muscle phosphoglycerate mutase deficiency revisited. Arch Neurol 2009;66:394–8.
18. Vissing J, Quistorff B, Haller RG. Effect of fuels on exercise capacity in muscle phosphoglycerate mutase deficiency. Arch Neurol 2005;62:1440–3.
19. Henry JG, Stevens SM. Neuronal ceroid lipofuscinosis in the amaurotic retardate: electron microscopic confirmation. Aust J Ophthalmol 1982;10:161–6.
20. Comi GP, Fortunato F, Lucchiari S, et al. Beta-enolase deficiency, a new metabolic myopathy of distal glycolysis. Ann Neurol 2001;50:202–7.

21. Kanno T, Sudo K, Takeuchi I, et al. Hereditary deficiency of lactate dehydrogenase M-subunit. Clin Chim Acta 1980;108:267–76.
22. Stojkovic T, Vissing J, Petit F, et al. Muscle glycogenosis due to phosphoglucomutase 1 deficiency. N Engl J Med 2009;361:425–7.
23. Rinaldo P, Matern D, Bennett MJ. Fatty acid oxidation disorders. Annu Rev Physiol 2002;64:477–502.
24. Vladutiu GD. The molecular diagnosis of metabolic myopathies. Neurol Clin 2000; 18:53–104.
25. Gillingham MB, Scott B, Elliott D, et al. Metabolic control during exercise with and without medium-chain triglycerides (MCT) in children with long-chain 3-hydroxy acyl-CoA dehydrogenase (LCHAD) or trifunctional protein (TFP) deficiency. Mol Genet Metab 2006;89:58–63.
26. Schymik I, Liebig M, Mueller M, et al. Pitfalls of neonatal screening for very-long-chain acyl-CoA dehydrogenase deficiency using tandem mass spectrometry. J Pediatr 2006;149:128–30.
27. Wilcken B. Fatty acid oxidation disorders: outcome and long-term prognosis. J Inherit Metab Dis 2010;33(5):501–6.
28. Gillingham MB, Weleber RG, Neuringer M, et al. Effect of optimal dietary therapy upon visual function in children with long-chain 3-hydroxyacyl CoA dehydrogenase and trifunctional protein deficiency. Mol Genet Metab 2005;86:124–33.
29. Scaglia F, Towbin JA, Craigen WJ, et al. Clinical spectrum, morbidity, and mortality in 113 pediatric patients with mitochondrial disease. Pediatrics 2004; 114:925–31.
30. Simon DK, Johns DR. Mitochondrial disorders: clinical and genetic features. Annu Rev Med 1999;50:111–27.
31. DiMauro S, Schon EA. Mitochondrial DNA mutations in human disease. Am J Med Genet 2001;106:18–26.
32. Alberio S, Mineri R, Tiranti V, et al. Depletion of mtDNA: syndromes and genes. Mitochondrion 2007;7:6–12.
33. Gempel K, Topaloglu H, Talim B, et al. The myopathic form of coenzyme Q10 deficiency is caused by mutations in the electron-transferring-flavoprotein dehydrogenase (ETFDH) gene. Brain 2007;130:2037–44.
34. Rodriguez MC, MacDonald JR, Mahoney DJ, et al. Beneficial effects of creatine, CoQ10, and lipoic acid in mitochondrial disorders. Muscle Nerve 2007;35: 235–42.

Drugs Causing Muscle Disease

Adam Mor, MD[a], Robert L. Wortmann, MD, MACR[b],
Hal J. Mitnick, MD[c], Michael H. Pillinger, MD[d],*

KEYWORDS

- Adverse drug reaction • Drug induced • Myopathy • Myalgias

Muscle weakness and/or myalgia is a common complaint among rheumatologic patients, and rheumatologists are aware of the importance of correctly diagnosing autoimmune myositis. However, while the differential diagnosis of muscle weakness should almost always also include drug effects, such effects may be difficult to identify. Many drugs can cause myopathies, and such myopathies may range widely from asymptomatic elevations in the serum creatine phosphokinase (CK) levels to severe myalgias, cramps, exercise intolerance, muscle weakness, and even rhabdomyolysis. Reviewing the literature frequently results in confusion because individual drugs may cause varying effects in different patients and imprecise terminologies are used to describe muscle pathology. In this article, some of the commonly used drugs that may induce myopathies, and the clinical syndromes, diagnosis, and management of these drug-induced myopathies are reviewed. For the convenience of the reader, the potential offending agents are segregated according to their major clinical indications.

DRUGS FOR CARDIOVASCULAR DISEASE
Statins and Other Lipid-Lowering Agents

The most prevalent drug-induced myopathies are those caused by lipid-lowering agents. 3-Hydroxy-3-methylglutaryl coenzyme A (HMG-CoA) reductase inhibitors (statins), fibric acid derivatives (fibrates), niacin, and ezetimibe may all cause myopathy in some patients.[1,2] However, it should be noted that the high prevalence of myotoxicities associated with these agents is not because of a large risk from their use but

The authors have nothing to disclose.
[a] Division of Rheumatology, Department of Medicine, New York University School of Medicine, 301 East 17th Street Room 1410, New York, NY 10003, USA
[b] Section of Rheumatology, Department of Medicine, Dartmouth Medical School and Dartmouth Hitchcock Medcial Center, Lebanon, NH 03756, USA
[c] Division of Rheumatology, Department of Medicine, New York University School of Medicine, 333 East 34th Street, New York, NY 10016, USA
[d] Division of Rheumatology, Department of Medicine, New York University School of Medicine, 301 East 14th Street Room 1410, New York, NY 10003, USA
* Corresponding author.
E-mail address: michael.pillinger@nyumc.org

rather because the use of such drugs is extremely common.[3] The typical syndrome of statin myopathies includes muscle pain and tenderness and weakness, with serum CK levels elevated at least 10-fold higher than the normal upper limit. By this definition, the incidence of statin-associated myopathy is no more than 11 per 100,000 person-years, with the incidence of statin-associated rhabdomyolysis being roughly 3.5 per 100,000 person-years.[4] Milder syndromes with lower CK levels may be more common. The combined use of fibrates and statins may increase the incidence of muscle diseases by as much as 10-fold. Statins vary vis-à-vis their ability to induce these effects; lovastatin, simvastatin, and atorvastatin (metabolized by cytochrome P450 [CYP]) carry a higher risk than pravastatin and fluvastatin.[5]

The effects of statins are quite variable. Some patients taking statins experience muscle symptoms despite normal CK levels, whereas others experience elevated CK levels without symptoms.[6–8] Caution must be exerted in interpreting isolated CK level elevations; in some studies, elevations less than 10 times the upper limit of the normal level have been documented to occur at equal rates irrespective of the patient taking a statin or a placebo.[4,9] Symptoms of statin-induced myopathy include myalgias, muscle tenderness, or weakness; localized ache or cramping may be characteristic features.[10] Tendon pain and nocturnal leg cramps may occur.[11,12] Weakness can occur in any muscle group but may be common in the proximal limbs and trunk.[6] Vigorous exercise is often poorly tolerated and can aggravate statin-induced myotoxicity.[13,14]

Typically, the onset of myopathy requires about 6 months of statin use to manifest.[7] Muscle symptoms usually, but not always, resolve after stopping the offending agent, but this may take some time.[13,14] Persistent symptoms after statin discontinuation may reflect the unmasking of a preexisting but previously unrecognized neuromuscular disorder, such as hypothyroidism, metabolic myopathy, myotonic dystrophy, spinal muscular atrophy, or inflammatory myositis.[15–19] In one study, 25 patients with proximal muscle weakness associated with statin use were found to have persistent weakness and elevated CK levels despite discontinuation of the offending drug. In these patients, muscle biopsy findings showed necrotizing myopathy. The lack of improvement after discontinuation of statins and the need for immunosuppressive therapy in treating these patients suggest an immune-mediated cause for this unusual statin-associated necrotizing myopathy.[20] In severe cases of myopathy, rhabdomyolysis may result in acute renal failure, disseminated intravascular coagulation, and death.[21,22]

Muscle biopsy specimens from patients with statin-associated myopathies may appear normal when viewed under light microscopy.[23] In other cases, biopsy specimens may show evidence of mitochondrial dysfunction, including ragged red fibers, and deficiency of cytochrome C oxidase on immunohistochemical analysis.[24] Fiber atrophy and lipid-laden vacuoles may also be observed.[13,24]

Myotoxicity from statins and other lipid-lowering agents occurs more frequently in the presence of higher serum drug levels. Thus, drug dose, drug-to-drug interactions, and renal and hepatic dysfunctions may all contribute to increased risk.[25–30] Older age and female sex also are independent risk factors for myopathy related to these agents.[31]

At the cellular level, molecular functions that increase intracellular statin concentrations may play a role in increased toxicity. For example, the transporter organic anion transporting polypeptide (OATP) promotes cellular uptake of statins and may promote toxicity.[31] In one in vitro study, OATP inhibition protected skeletal myofibers against statin-induced toxicity.[32] At the genetic level, specific polymorphisms of SLCO1B1 (the OATP gene) have been shown to affect transporter activity, with potential implications for statin myotoxic susceptibility. In another study, polymorphisms in the gene for ABCB1, an efflux transporter, were associated with altered risk for simvastatin-related myopathy.[31,32]

Myotoxicity risk may be increased when more than one class of lipid-lowering agents are administered together. Gemfibrozil (but not fenofibrate) inhibits statin elimination.[28] Use of a statin together with niacin is associated with a rare but increased risk of rhabdomyolysis.[29] Anecdotal reports of myopathy attributed to the combination of statin and ezetimibe have been reported, but these reports are not supported by pooled data from clinical trials, including 14,471 patients.[32]

Because most statins are metabolized by the hepatic CYP system, coadministration of such agents with another drug that is metabolized by the CYP system can result in drug-to-drug interactions. Drugs that are metabolized by the alternative liver isoenzyme CYP3A4 (cyclosporine, erythromycin, azole antifungals, diltiazem, ritonavir, and nefazodone) can also increase the risk of statin-induced myotoxicity. Metabolism of fluvastatin can be impaired by coadministration of other CYP2C9 substrates, such as diclofenac, warfarin, or tolbutamide.[33]

The mechanisms through which lipid-lowering agents cause myotoxicity are not well established. Proposed mechanisms include alterations to membranes and/or mitochondria. HMG-CoA reductase inhibition (the major statin effect) may affect the function of transfer RNAs, glycoproteins, the electron transport chain, and proteins that depend on HMG-CoA reductase for posttranslational modification.[34] Decreases in ubiquinone expression have been described in the muscles of some patients, but it is unknown whether this decrease may be a cause or consequence of statin use.[13,32,35] Some patients with statin-induced myopathy have been found to have abnormalities in muscle carnitine levels.[36] Hanai and colleagues[37] reported that lovastatin induced the expression of atrogin-1, a key gene involved in human skeletal muscle atrophy. Induction of atrogin-1 by statins was accompanied by morphologic changes and muscle fiber damage, an effect that was similar to knocking down HMG-CoA reductase, suggesting that atrogin-1 may be a mediator of the muscle damage induced by statins. In a follow-up study, the investigators reported that lovastatin-induced atrogin-1 expression and muscle damage could be prevented in the presence of geranylgeranylation inhibitors. These findings support the concept that dysfunction of small GTP-binding proteins leads to statin-induced muscle damage.[38]

Management of severe myopathy induced by lipid-lowering drugs is straightforward and requires drug discontinuation and, if necessary, hospital admission to manage rhabdomyolysis. Management is less clear for milder cases and may range from close monitoring to lowering or discontinuing the agent or switching to a different statin or other lipid-lowering agent; some reports suggest a possible benefit from coenzyme Q10 supplementation.[39–44]

Antiarrhythmic Agents

Reports suggest that several antiarrhythmic agents may also cause muscle problems. Amiodarone may rarely cause both proximal and distal muscle weakness, as well as distal sensory loss, tremor, and ataxia.[45] These toxicities are more common in patients with chronic kidney disease. Serum CK levels may be increased. Electromyography (EMG) results reveal positive sharp waves, fibrillation potentials, and early recruitment of motor unit action potentials in proximal muscles versus polyphasic action potentials of large amplitude and long duration in distal muscles.[46] Autophagic vacuoles containing myeloid inclusions and debris are found on biopsy analysis. Amiodarone-induced myopathy gradually resolves after therapy is discontinued. Clinicians should keep in mind, however, that amiodarone can also induce hypothyroidism with resulting muscle sequelae that can confuse the clinical picture.[47]

Procainamide can cause myalgias and proximal muscle weakness, often as part of a drug-induced lupus syndrome.[48,49] Serum CK levels are increased, and EMG findings are consistent with those of inflammatory myopathy. Labetalol may sometimes induce an acute or insidious onset of proximal muscle weakness or myalgias.[50] Other cardioactive drugs that may rarely cause myopathy after prolonged administration include aminocaproic acid, warfarin, and calcium channel antagonists such as diltiazem.[44]

RHEUMATOLOGIC DRUGS
Corticosteroids

Corticosteroid myopathy is relatively common, owing to both the toxicity of these agents and the frequency with which they are prescribed. In steroid myopathy, weakness (especially proximal muscle weakness) typically comes on insidiously, and CK levels are normal. Corticosteroid myopathy usually is seen in the setting of chronic use of high doses of steroids, especially multiple doses per day. However, corticosteroid myopathy may come on rapidly (days) and even when low doses are used.[51] Some data suggest that fluorinated glucocorticoids (triamcinolone, betamethasone, and dexamethasone) may carry a lower risk.[52,53] In contrast, according to the more recent literature, side effects occur more frequently and are worse after treatment with fluorinated steroids than after treatment with nonfluorinated steroids.[54] Respiratory muscles can occasionally be involved.[55,56] Necrotizing myopathy is a very rare consequence of steroid use, and high-dose intravenous corticosteroids have been reported to cause an acute quadriplegic state.[57]

As in the case of statins, the mechanisms through which steroids act on the muscle remain uncertain. Proposed hypotheses include alterations in muscle protein synthesis and/or degradation, altered muscle metabolism, reduced sarcolemmal excitability, and corticosteroid-induced hypokalemia.[58–60] EMG findings are typically normal, and muscle biopsy results either are normal or show nonspecific type 2 fiber atrophy.[61,62] Whenever possible, treatment of corticosteroid-induced myopathy should include discontinuation of the offending agent. If not possible, attempts should be made to reduce the dosage to a physiologic dose.[63] Recovery usually occurs with discontinuation of the steroid but may take an extended period, especially if usage has been long-term.[51,64] Rapid withdrawal of chronically used steroids may itself result in hypoadrenalism, including weakness.

Colchicine

Colchicine can cause multiple neuromuscular complications. Generalized myopathy and painful neuromyopathy are the most common complications and may appear early after initiation or after months of therapy.[33,65,66] Chronic kidney disease or diuretic use increases the risk.[33] Colchicine is metabolized by the CYP3A4 system, and coadministration of any drug that is metabolized by CYP3A4 can precipitate colchicine myopathy.[67] Concomitant cyclosporine or clarithromycin use increases the risk of colchicine-induced rhabdomyolysis.[33,67]

Colchicine myopathy is believed to result from colchicine's ability to inhibit microtubule polymerization, as well as changes in the expression of dopaminergic receptors.[68] Patients may be symptomatic or asymptomatic, with CK level elevations from minimal to 100 times normal. EMG and nerve conduction studies may show both neuropathic and myopathic changes, including prolonged distal motor and sensory latencies.[69] Muscle biopsy specimens show autophagic vacuoles that stain positively for acid phosphatase.[69] Electron microscopy may show colchicine bodies (clumps of chromatin in the nuclei of hepatocytes).[70] Nerve biopsy rarely needs to be performed, but its results may show axonal neuropathy. Treatment is discontinuation of colchicine, which generally results in complete resolution, although this may take months.

Chloroquines

Chloroquine and related agents may cause myopathy that is typically painless, slowly progressive, and typically more pronounced proximally and in the lower extremities. Severe cases may present as myasthenia-like syndrome or myotonia.[71,72] Neuropathy may occur uncommonly, and cardiomyopathy has been reported. Onset typically occurs months to years after start of treatment.[73] Serum CK levels are elevated, and EMG shows myopathic changes of increased insertional activity with positive waves, fibrillations, and other characteristic changes.[74] Muscle biopsy specimens show vacuoles containing acid phosphatase and, on electron microscopy, concentric lamellar debris and curvilinear bodies.[75]

The pathologic mechanism of chloroquine myopathy is thought to derive from the ability of these agents to form drug-lipid complexes in cellular membranes, resulting in the accumulation of autophagic vacuoles.[76,77] This model has been confirmed in rats administered chloroquine (50 mg/kg twice daily for 8 weeks), resulting in myopathy characterized by accumulation of autophagic vacuoles.[78] In patients, discontinuation of the chloroquine results in improvement over months.[79] Animal studies suggest that administration of the cysteine proteinase inhibitor EST (loxistation) may hasten resolution.[80]

Other Immunomodulatory Agents

With persistent use, cyclosporine and tacrolimus may induce myalgias, cramps, proximal muscle weakness, and, in some cases, rhabdomyolysis.[81–84] EMG shows fibrillation potentials, sharp positive waves, and myotonic potentials, and atrophy and necrosis may be seen in muscle biopsy specimens.[85] The risk of myopathy from these drugs is exacerbated by the concurrent use of a statin or colchicine.[70] Because these drugs may occasionally be used in inflammatory myositis, their potential adverse effects on the muscle may complicate the clinical picture.[86]

D-Penicillamine can induce polymyositis or dermatomyositis in a small percentage of patients.[87] Azathioprine has been rarely associated with rhabdomyolysis.[88] Myokymia (arrhythmic rippling of muscles) is a rare complication of gold therapy.[89] In one study, infliximab was associated with clinical worsening of myositis.[90] Cases of myositis in the setting of interferon use have been reported and improve with treatment discontinuation.[44,91,92]

INFECTIOUS DISEASE DRUGS
Antiviral Agents

Many antiviral agents can cause myopathy. The most common offending agent is zidovudine, which causes myalgias and proximal muscle weakness.[93–95] Other nucleoside analogue reverse transcriptase inhibitors (didanosine, lamivudine, and zalcitabine) can have similar effects.[96–98] Serum CK levels are typically normal or slightly elevated. EMG changes, seen in proximal muscles, may include insertional activity with sharp waves and fibrillation potentials, early recruitment of polyphasic action potentials, and complex repetitive discharges.[99,100] However, these findings must be differentiated from primary human immunodeficiency virus–associated myopathy.[100] Histologic examination of reverse transcriptase–associated myopathy shows signs of mitochondrial involvement, including ragged red fibers.[94,101] Necrosis, microvacuoles, cytoplasmic bodies, and nemaline rods may all be seen.[94,95] Proposed mechanisms of antiretroviral myopathy include the effects of oxidative stress, inhibition of mitochondrial energetics, L-carnitine depletion, and apoptosis.[102] Tenofovir and ritonavir have been reported to cause rhabdomyolysis, particularly in patients taking another myopathy-inducing drug.[103,104]

Antifungal and Antibacterial Agents

Ketoconazole and itraconazole have been reported to cause myopathy or rhabdomyolysis in conjunction with simultaneous statin use.[105,106] Rifampin use had been associated with a proximal myopathy with normal EMG findings and CK levels.[107] Myalgias and malignant hyperthermia have been associated with quinolone derivatives, as also described earlier.[108,109]

ONCOLOGY DRUGS

Vincristine, an agent that disrupts microtubule polymerization, may cause proximal muscle weakness and myalgias, with denervation and necrosis observed on biopsy findings.[110] Imatinib mesylate causes myalgias in up to 50% of patients, with a single case report of imatinib-associated polymyositis.[111] Cardiotoxicity and dermatomyositis-like disease have also been reported.[112] An inflammatory myopathy has been reported in association with the use of leuprolide acetate.[113] Cases of rhabdomyolysis have been reported in patients taking 5-azacytidine, cytarabine, and the combination of cyclophosphamide and mitoxantrone.[114,115]

All-trans retinoic acid is used to treat patients with acute promyelocytic leukemia. Cases of new-onset myopathy after receiving this agent have been reported. The condition can manifest as myalgia, stiffness, and, in rare cases, rhabdomyolysis. CK levels have been found to be elevated, occasionally by up to 100 times the normal value, particularly in patients performing physical exercise.[116] Inflammatory myositis has been described as well. This adverse reaction is noticeable for fever, myalgia, arthralgia, and Sweet syndrome, accompanied by distinct magnetic resonance imaging findings involving the lower extremity musculature. Treatment consists of discontinuation of the offending drug and, often, high-dose steroids.[117]

GASTROINTESTINAL DRUGS

In rare instances, omeprazole is associated with a lower extremity neuromyopathy, including proximal weakness, myalgias, and paresthesias.[118] Serum CK levels are increased, and nerve conduction studies may show an axonal sensorimotor neuropathy. Other proton pump inhibitors have also been associated with myopathy. Polymyositis in the setting of proton pump inhibitor use has been reported; most cases resolved with drug discontinuation.[119] Patients taking cimetidine or ranitidine may also occasionally experience myalgias, cramps, weakness or myokymia, and possibly polymyositis.[120,121]

NEUROLOGIC AND PSYCHIATRIC DRUGS

Myalgias and weakness sometimes occur in the setting of phenytoin hypersensitivity responses.[122,123] CK level elevations are typical, and muscle histology reveals degenerating and regenerating fibers. Patients improve with drug discontinuation, with or without the addition of glucocorticoids. Valproic acid can induce carnitine deficiency, resulting in limb-girdle weakness with EMG changes.[124] Patients with lipid storage disorders or carnitine palmitoyltransferase deficiency may be particularly susceptible.[125,126] Levodopa has also been associated with myositis.[110] In up to 10% of patients receiving the antipsychotics clozapine, risperidone, melperone, olanzapine, loxapine, or haloperidol, CK levels may be elevated, sometimes to moderately high levels. The myopathic effects of antipsychotics may be related to blockade of 5-hydroxytryptamine receptors in the sarcolemma.[44]

Malignant hyperthermia is characterized by muscle rigidity, fever, and myoglobinuria. Most cases are a rare consequence of treatment with depolarizing muscle relaxants (eg, succinylcholine) or inhaled anesthetics (eg, halothane). Tricyclic antidepressants and monamine oxidase inhibitors have also been rarely implicated.[33] Individuals with preexisting muscular dystrophy may be particularly susceptible.[127] More than half of the patients experiencing malignant hyperthermia had previously undergone anesthesia without a problem.[128] The condition is associated with the autosomal dominant inheritance of one of several different genes, including the genes for the ryanodine receptor, the dihydropyridine-sensitive L-type voltage-dependent calcium channel gene, and the calcium channel subunit CACNA 2.[33] These mutations cause excessive calcium release from the sarcoplasmic reticulum, resulting in persistent muscle contraction. Serum CK levels are normal or mildly elevated in asymptomatic susceptible individuals but increase dramatically during attacks.

SUMMARY

The spectrum of drug-induced myopathies ranges from asymptomatic serum CK level elevations to severe rhabdomyolysis. Although some drugs predictably cause myopathy, virtually any medication may rarely have this effect. In most cases, the pathophysiology of drug-induced myopathy is poorly understood, with much to be learned about the ways in which muscles can fail. Drug-induced myopathy should be considered in the setting of de novo onset of muscle symptoms, particularly when no other recognizable cause of myopathy is identified. In most cases, drug-induced myopathy occurs shortly after administering the agent, but in some cases, myopathy can develop after long-term use. When a drug-related myopathy is suspected, the purported offending agent should be withdrawn or reduced if possible. Although in some cases the disease may persist despite drug discontinuation, early diagnosis and cessation of treatment improves the chances of a more rapid and complete resolution.

REFERENCES

1. Havranek JM, Wolfsen AR, Warnke GA, et al. Monotherapy with ezetimibe causing myopathy. Am J Med 2006;119:285–6.
2. Simard C, Poirier P. Ezetimibe-associated myopathy in monotherapy and in combination with a 3-hydroxy-3-methylglutaryl coenzyme A reductase inhibitor. Can J Cardiol 2006;22:141–4.
3. Silva MA, Swanson AC, Gandhi PJ, et al. Statin-related adverse events: a meta-analysis. Clin Ther 2006;28:26–35.
4. Law M, Rudnicka AR. Statin safety: a systematic review. Am J Cardiol 2006;97: 52–60.
5. Kobayashi M, Chisaki I, Narumi K, et al. Association between risk of myopathy and cholesterol-lowering effect: a comparison of all statins. Life Sci 2008;82: 969–75.

6. Phillips PS, Haas RH, Bannykh S, et al. Statin-associated myopathy with normal creatine kinase levels. Ann Intern Med 2002;137:581–5.
7. Hansen KE, Hildebrand JP, Ferguson EE, et al. Outcomes in 45 patients with statin-associated myopathy. Arch Intern Med 2005;165:2671–6.
8. Baker SK, Tarnopolsky MA. Statin-associated neuromyotoxicity. Drugs Today (Barc) 2005;41:267–93.
9. Mor A, Pillinger MH, Wortmann RL, et al. Drug-induced arthritic and connective tissue disorders. Semin Arthritis Rheum 2008;38:249–64.
10. Sinzinger H, Wolfram R, Peskar BA. Muscular side effects of statins. J Cardiovasc Pharmacol 2002;40:163–71.
11. Bennett WE, Drake AJ 3rd, Shakir K. Reversible myopathy after statin therapy in patients with normal creatine kinase levels. Ann Intern Med 2003;138:436–7.
12. Franc S, Dejager S, Bruckert E, et al. A comprehensive description of muscle symptoms associated with lipid-lowering drugs. Cardiovasc Drugs Ther 2003; 17:459–65.
13. Vladutiu GD, Simmons Z, Isackson PJ, et al. Genetic risk factors associated with lipid-lowering drug-induced myopathies. Muscle Nerve 2006;34:153–62.
14. Phillips PS, Phillips CT, Sullivan MJ, et al. Statin myotoxicity is associated with changes in the cardiopulmonary function. Atherosclerosis 2004;177:183–8.
15. Fauchais AL, Iba Ba J, Maurage P, et al. Polymyositis induced or associated with lipid-lowering drugs: five cases. Rev Med Interne 2004;25:294–8.
16. Vasconcelos OM, Campbell WW. Dermatomyositis-like syndrome and HMG-CoA reductase inhibitor (statin) intake. Muscle Nerve 2004;30:803–7.
17. Rando LP, Cording SA, Newnham HH. Successful reintroduction of statin therapy after myositis: was there another cause? Med J Aust 2004;180:472–3.
18. Tsivgoulis G, Spengos K, Karandreas N, et al. Presymptomatic neuromuscular disorders disclosed following statin treatment. Arch Intern Med 2006;166: 1519–24.
19. Diaczok BJ, Shali R. Statins unmasking a mitochondrial myopathy: a case report and proposed mechanism of disease. South Med J 2003;96:318–20.
20. Grable-Esposito P, Katzberg HD, Greenberg SA, et al. Immune-mediated necrotizing myopathy associated with statins. Muscle Nerve 2010;41:185–90.
21. Hazin R, Abuzetun JY, Suker M, et al. Rhabdomyolysis induced by simvastatin-fluconazole combination. J Natl Med Assoc 2008;100:444–6.
22. Bays H. Statin safety: an overview and assessment of the data—2005. Am J Cardiol 2006;97:6–26.
23. Lamperti C, Naini AB, Lucchini V, et al. Muscle coenzyme Q10 level in statin-related myopathy. Arch Neurol 2005;62:1709–12.
24. Gambelli S, Dotti MT, Malandrini A, et al. Mitochondrial alterations in muscle biopsies of patients on statin therapy. J Submicrosc Cytol Pathol 2004;36: 85–9.
25. Pfeffer MA, Keech A, Sacks FM, et al. Safety and tolerability of pravastatin in long-term clinical trials: Prospective Pravastatin Pooling (PPP) Project. Circulation 2002;105:2341–6.
26. Graham DJ, Staffa JA, Shatin D, et al. Incidence of hospitalized rhabdomyolysis in patients treated with lipid-lowering drugs. JAMA 2004;292:2585–90.
27. Chang JT, Staffa JA, Parks M, et al. Rhabdomyolysis with HMG-CoA reductase inhibitors and gemfibrozil combination therapy. Pharmacoepidemiol Drug Saf 2004;13:417–26.
28. Jones PH, Davidson MH. Reporting rate of rhabdomyolysis with fenofibrate plus statin versus gemfibrozil plus any statin. Am J Cardiol 2005;95:120–2.

29. Shek A, Ferrill JM. Statin-fibrate combination therapy. Ann Pharmacother 2001; 35:908–17.
30. Omar MA, Wilson JP, Cox TS. Rhabdomyolysis and HMG-CoA reductase inhibitors. Ann Pharmacother 2001;35:1096–107.
31. Peters BJM, Klungel OH, Visseren FL, et al. Pharmacogenomic insights into treatment and management of statin-induced myopathy. Genome Med 2009; 1:1201–4.
32. Yiannis SC, Konstantinos CK, Gesthimani M, et al. Risk factors and drug interactions predisposing to statin-induced myopathy. Drug Saf 2010;33:171–87.
33. Mor A, Mitnick HJ, Pillinger MH, et al. Drug-induced myopathies. Bull NYU Hosp Jt Dis 2009;67:358–69.
34. Flint OP, Masters BA, Gregg RE, et al. HMG-CoA reductase inhibitor-induced myotoxicity: pravastatin and lovastatin inhibit the geranylgeranylation of low-molecular-weight proteins in neonatal rat muscle cell culture. Toxicol Appl Pharmacol 1997;145:99–110.
35. Schaefer WH, Lawrence JW, Loughlin AF, et al. Evaluation of ubiquinone concentration and mitochondrial function relative to cerivastatin-induced skeletal myopathy in rats. Toxical Appl Pharmacol 2004;194:10–23.
36. Paiva H, Thelen KM, Van Coster R, et al. High-dose statins and skeletal muscle metabolism in humans: a randomized, controlled trial. Clin Pharmacol Ther 2005;78:60–8.
37. Hanai J, Cao P, Tanksale P, et al. The muscle-specific ubiquitin ligase atrogin-1/MAFbx mediates statin-induced muscle toxicity. J Clin Invest 2007;117: 3940–51.
38. Cao P, Hanai J, Tanksale P, et al. Statin-induced muscle damage and atrogin-1 induction is the result of a geranylgeranylation defect. FASEB J 2009;23: 2844–54.
39. Seehusen DA, Asplund CA, Johnson DR, et al. Primary evaluation and management of statin therapy complications. South Med J 2006;99:250–6.
40. Antons KA, Williams CD, Baker SK, et al. Clinical perspectives of statin-induced rhabdomyolysis. Am J Med 2006;119:400–9.
41. Koumis T, Nathan JP, Rosenberg JM, et al. Strategies for the prevention and treatment of statin-induced myopathy: is there a role for ubiquinone supplementation? Am J Health Syst Pharm 2004;61:515–9.
42. Kelly P, Vasu S, Gelato M, et al. Coenzyme Q10 improves myopathic pain in statin treated patients. J Am Coll Cardiol 2005;45:3.
43. Campbell WW. Statin myopathy: the iceberg or its tip? Muscle Nerve 2006;34: 387–90.
44. Dalakas MC. Toxic and drug-induced myopathies. J Neurol Neurosurg Psychiatry 2009;80:832–8.
45. Fernando Roth R, Itabashi H, Louie J, et al. Amiodarone toxicity: myopathy and neuropathy. Am Heart J 1990;119:1223–5.
46. Meier C, Kauer B, Muller U, et al. Neuromyopathy during chronic amiodarone treatment. A case report. J Neurol 1979;220:231–9.
47. Merz T, Fuller SH. Elevated serum transaminase levels resulting from concomitant use of rosuvastatin and amiodarone. Am J Health Syst Pharm 2007;64: 1818–21.
48. Miller CD, Oleshansky MA, Gibson KF, et al. Procainamide-induced myasthenia-like weakness and dysphagia. Ther Drug Monit 1993;15:251–4.
49. Lewis CA, Boheimer N, Rose P, et al. Myopathy after short term administration of procainamide. Br Med J 1986;292:593–4.

50. Willis JK, Tilton AH, Harkin JC, et al. Reversible myopathy due to labetalol. Pediatr Neurol 1990;6:275–6.
51. Kissil JT, Mendell JR. The endocrine myopathies. In: Rowland LP, DiMauro S, editors. Handbook of clinical neurology, vol. 18. Amsterdam (Netherlands): Elsevier Science Publishers; 1992. p. 527–51.
52. Dubois EL. Triamcinolone in the treatment of systemic lupus erythematosus. JAMA 1958;167:1590–9.
53. Afifi AK, Bergman RA, Harvey JC. Steroid myopathy. Clinical, histological, and cytologic observations. Johns Hopkins Med J 1968;123:158–74.
54. van Balkom RH, van der Heijden HF, van Herwaarden CL, et al. Corticosteroid-induced myopathy of the respiratory muscles. Neth J Med 1994;45:114–22.
55. Decramer M, de Bock V, Dom R. Functional and histologic picture of steroid-induced myopathy in chronic obstructive pulmonary disease. Am J Respir Crit Care Med 1996;153:1958–64.
56. Yamaguchi M, Niimi A, Minakuchi M, et al. Corticosteroid-induced myopathy mimicking therapy-resistant asthma. Ann Allergy Asthma Immunol 2007;99: 371–4.
57. Hanson P, Dive A, Brucher JM, et al. Acute corticosteroid myopathy in intensive care patients. Muscle Nerve 1997;20:1371–80.
58. Pacy PJ, Halliday D. Muscle protein synthesis in steroid-induced proximal myopathy: a case report. Muscle Nerve 1989;12:378–81.
59. Oshima Y, Kuroda Y, Kunishige M, et al. Oxidative stress-associated mitochondrial dysfunction in corticosteroid-treated muscle cells. Muscle Nerve 2004;30: 49–54.
60. Powell RJ. Steroid and hypokalemic myopathy after corticosteroids for ulcerative colitis. Am J Gastroenterol 1969;52:425–32.
61. Askari A, Vignos PJ, Moskowitz RW. Steroid myopathy in connective tissue disease. Am J Med 1976;61:485–92.
62. Khaleeli AA, Edwards RHT, Gohil K, et al. Corticosteroid myopathy: a clinical and pathological study. Clin Endocrinol (Oxf) 1983;18:155–66.
63. Horber FF, Scheidegger JR, Grunwig BE, et al. Evidence that prednisone-induced myopathy is reversed by physical training. J Clin Endocrinol Metab 1985;61:83–8.
64. Faludi G, Gotlieb J, Meyers J. Factors influencing the development of steroid-induced myopathies. Ann N Y Acad Sci 1966;138:62–72.
65. Riggs JE, Schochet SS Jr, Gutmann L, et al. Chronic human colchicine neuropathy and myopathy. Arch Neurol 1986;43:521–3.
66. Schiff D, Drislane FW. Rapid-onset colchicine myoneuropathy. Arthritis Rheum 1992;35:1535–6.
67. McKinnell J, Tayek JA. Short term treatment with clarithromycin resulting in colchicine-induced rhabdomyolysis. J Clin Rheumatol 2009;15:303–5.
68. Jiang Q, Yan Z, Feng J. Neurotrophic factors stabilize microtubules and protect against rotenone toxicity on dopaminergic neurons. J Biol Chem 2006;281: 29391–400.
69. Kuncl RW, Cornblath DR, Avila O, et al. Electrodiagnosis of human colchicine myoneuropathy. Muscle Nerve 1989;12:360–4.
70. Sundov Z, Nincevic Z, Definis-Gojanovic M, et al. Fatal colchicine poisoning by accidental ingestion of meadow saffron-case report. Forensic Sci Int 2004;149: 253–6.
71. Sghirlanzoni A, Mantegazza R, Mora M, et al. Chloroquine myopathy and myasthenia-like syndrome. Muscle Nerve 1988;11:114–9.

72. Kwiecinski H. Myotonia induced by chemical agents. Crit Rev Toxicol 1981;90: 287–99.
73. Stein M, Bell MJ, Ang LC. Hydroxychloroquine neuromyotoxicity. J Rheumatol 2000;27:2927–31.
74. Estes ML, Ewing-Wilson D, Chou SM, et al. Chloroquine neuromyotoxicity. Clinical and pathologic perspective. Am J Med 1987;82:447–55.
75. Casado E, Gratacos J, Tolosa C, et al. Antimalarial myopathy: an underdiagnosed complication? Prospective longitudinal study of 119 patients. Ann Rheum Dis 2006;65:385–90.
76. Avina-Zubieta JA, Johnson ES, Suarez-Almazor ME, et al. Incidence of myopathy in patients treated with antimalarials. A report of three cases and a review of the literature. Br J Rheumatol 1995;34:166–70.
77. Walsh RJ, Amato AA. Toxic myopathies. Neurol Clin 2005;23:397–428.
78. Kimura N, Kumamoto T, Kawamura Y, et al. Expression of autophagy-associated genes in skeletal muscle: an experimental model of chloroquine-induced myopathy. Pathobiology 2007;74:169–76.
79. Becerra-Cuñat JL, Coll-Cantí J, Gelpí-Mantius E, et al. Chloroquine-induced myopathy and neuropathy: progressive tetraparesis with areflexia that simulates a polyradiculoneuropathy. Two case reports. Rev Neurol 2003;36:523–6.
80. Sugita H, Higuchi I, Sano M, et al. Trial of a cysteine proteinase inhibitor, EST, in experimental chloroquine myopathy in rats. Muscle Nerve 1987;10:516–23.
81. Grezard O, Lebranchu Y, Birmele B, et al. Cyclosporin-induced muscular toxicity. Lancet 1990;335:177.
82. Noppen M, Velkeniers B, Dierckx R, et al. Cyclosporine and myopathy. Ann Intern Med 1987;107:945–6.
83. Norman DJ, Illingworth DR, Munson J, et al. Myolysis and acute renal failure in a heart-transplant recipient receiving lovastatin. N Engl J Med 1988;318:46–7.
84. Atkison P, Joubert G, Barron A, et al. Hypertrophic cardiomyopathy associated with tacrolimus in paediatric transplant patients. Lancet 1995;345:894–6.
85. Costigan DA. Acquired myotonia, weakness and vacuolar myopathy secondary to cyclosporine. Muscle Nerve 1989;12:761.
86. Martín NA, Modesto CC, Arnal GC, et al. Efficacy of tacrolimus (FK-506) in the treatment of recalcitrant juvenile dermatomyositis: study of 6 cases. Med Clin (Barc) 2006;127:697–701.
87. Takahashi K, Ogita T, Okudaira H, et al. D-penicillamine-induced polymyositis in patients with rheumatoid arthritis. Arthritis Rheum 1986;29:560–4.
88. Compton MR, Crosby DL. Rhabdomyolysis associated with azathioprine hypersensitivity syndrome. Arch Dermatol 1996;132:1254–5.
89. Caldron PH, Wilbourn AJ, Bravo EE, et al. Gold myokymia syndrome. A rare toxic manifestation of chrysotherapy. Cleve Clin J Med 1987;54:225–8.
90. Dastmalchi M, Grundtman C, Alexanderson H, et al. A high incidence of disease flares in an open pilot study of infliximab in patients with refractory inflammatory myopathies. Ann Rheum Dis 2008;67:1670–7.
91. Dietrich LL, Bridges AJ, Albertini MR. Dermatomyositis after interferon alpha treatment. Med Oncol 2000;17:64–9.
92. Hengstman GJ, Vogels OJ, ter Laak HJ, et al. Myositis during long-term interferon-alpha treatment. Neurology 2000;54:2186.
93. Bessen LJ, Greene JB, Louie E, et al. Severe polymyositis-like syndrome associated with zidovudine therapy of AIDS and ARC. N Engl J Med 1988;318:708.
94. Dalakas MC, Illa I, Pezeshkpour GH, et al. Mitochondrial myopathy caused by long-term zidovudine therapy. N Engl J Med 1990;322:1098–105.

95. Grau JM, Masanes F, Pedrol E, et al. Human immunodeficiency virus type 1 infection and myopathy: clinical relevance of zidovudine therapy. Ann Neurol 1993;34:206–11.
96. Benbrik E, Chariot P, Bonavaud S, et al. Cellular and mitochondrial toxicity of zidovudine (AZT), didanosine (ddI) and zalcitabine (ddC) on cultured human muscle cells. J Neurol Sci 1997;149:19–25.
97. Pedrol E, Masanes F, Fernandez-Sola J, et al. Lack of muscle toxicity with didanosine (ddI). Clinical and experimental studies. J Neurol Sci 1996;138:42–8.
98. Simpson DM, Katzenstein DA, Hughes MD, et al. Neuromuscular function in HIV infection: analysis of a placebo-controlled combination antiretroviral trial. AIDS Clinical Group 175/801 Study Team. AIDS 1998;12:2425–32.
99. Simpson DM, Bender AN. Human immunodeficiency virus-associated myopathy: analysis of 11 patients. Ann Neurol 1988;24:79–84.
100. Simpson DM, Citak KA, Godfrey E, et al. Myopathies associated with human immunodeficiency virus and zidovudine: can their effects be distinguished? Neurology 1993;43:971–6.
101. Côté HCF, Brumme ZL, Craib KJP, et al. Changes in mitochondrial DNA as a marker of nucleoside toxicity in HIV-infected patients. N Engl J Med 2002; 346:811–20.
102. Scruggs ER, Dirks Naylor AJ. Mechanisms of zidovudine-induced mitochondrial toxicity and myopathy. Pharmacology 2008;82:83–8.
103. Callens S, De Roo A, Colebunders R. Fanconi-like syndrome and rhabdomyolysis in a person with HIV infection on highly active antiretroviral treatment including tenofovir. J Infect 2003;47:262–3.
104. Mah Ming JB, Gill MJ. Drug-induced rhabdomyolysis after concomitant use of clarithromycin, atorvastatin, lopinavir/ritonavir in a patient with HIV. AIDS Patient Care STDS 2003;17:207–10.
105. Gilad R, Lampl Y. Rhabdomyolysis induced by simvastatin and ketoconazole treatment. Clin Neuropharmacol 1999;22:295–7.
106. Lees RS, Lees AM. Rhabdomyolysis from the coadministration of lovastatin and the antifungal agent itraconazole. N Engl J Med 1995;333:664–5.
107. Jenkins P, Emerson PA. Myopathy induced by rifampicin. Br Med J 1981;283: 105–6.
108. Guis S, Bendahan D, Kozak-Ribbens G, et al. Investigation of fluoroquinolone-induced myalgia using magnetic resonance spectroscopy and in vitro contracture tests. Arthritis Rheum 2002;46:774–8.
109. Guis S, Jouglard J, Kozak-Ribbens G, et al. Malignant hyperthermia susceptibility revealed by myalgia and rhabdomyolysis during fluoroquinolone treatment. J Rheumatol 2001;28:1405–6.
110. Le Quintrec JS, Le Quintrec JL. Drug-induced myopathies. Baillieres Clin Rheumatol 1991;5:21–38.
111. Srinivasan J, Wu C, Amato AA. Inflammatory myopathy associated with imatinib therapy. J Clin Neuromuscul Dis 2004;5:119–21.
112. Kuwano Y, Asahina A, Watanabe R, et al. Heliotrope-like eruption mimicking dermatomyositis in a patient treated with imatinib mesylate for chronic myeloid leukemia. Int J Dermatol 2006;45:1249–51.
113. Crayton H, Bohlmann T, Sufit R, et al. Drug induced polymyositis secondary to leuprolide acetate (Lupron) therapy for prostate carcinoma. Clin Exp Rheumatol 1991;9:935–8.
114. Koeffler HP, Haskell CM. Rhabdomyolysis as a complication of 5-azacytidine. Cancer Treat Rep 1978;62:573–4.

115. Levy RJ, Sparano JA, Khan G. Rhabdomyolysis: an unusual complication of cytotoxic chemotherapy. Med Oncol 1995;12:219–22.

116. Chroni E, Monastirli A, Tsambaos D. Neuromuscular adverse effects associated with systemic retinoid dermatotherapy: monitoring and treatment algorithm for clinicians. Drug Saf 2010;33:25–34.

117. Yu W, Burns CM. All-trans retinoic acid-induced focal myositis, synovitis, and mononeuritis. J Clin Rheumatol 2009;15:358–60.

118. Faucheux JM, Tournebize P, Viguier A, et al. Neuromyopathy secondary to omeprazole treatment. Muscle Nerve 1998;21:261–2.

119. Clark DW, Strandell J. Myopathy including polymyositis: a likely class adverse effect of proton pump inhibitors? Eur J Clin Pharmacol 2006;62:473–9.

120. Hawkins RA, Eckhoff PJ Jr, MacCarter DK, et al. Cimetidine and polymyositis. N Engl J Med 1983;309:187–8.

121. Pelletier A, Ekert S, Hauw JJ, et al. Inflammatory myopathy during ranitidine therapy. J Rheumatol 1993;20:1453–4.

122. Harney J, Glasberg MR. Myopathy and hypersensitivity to phenytoin. Neurology 1983;33:790–1.

123. Tun NZ, Andermann F, Carpenter S, et al. Antiepileptic drug myopathy. Neurology 1994;44:777–8.

124. Sangeeta P. Sodium valproate-induced skeletal myopathy. Indian J Pediatr 2005;72:243–4.

125. Papadimitriou A, Servidei S. Late onset lipid storage myopathy due to multiple acyl CoA dehydrogenase deficiency triggered by valproate. Neuromuscul Disord 1991;1:247–52.

126. Kottlors M, Jaksch M, Ketelsen UP, et al. Valproic acid triggers acute rhabdomyolysis in a carnitine palmitoyltransferase type II deficiency. Neuromuscul Disord 2001;11:757–9.

127. Sethna RL, Rockoff MA, Worthen HM, et al. Anesthesia-related complications in children with Duchenne muscular dystrophy. Anethesiology 1988;68:462–5.

128. Griggs RC, Mendell JR, Miller RG. Myopathies of systemic disease. Evaluation and treatment of myopathies. Philadelphia: FA Davis; 1995. p. 355–85.

Muscular Dystrophies and Neurologic Diseases that Present as Myopathy

Dianna Quan, MD

KEYWORDS

• Muscular dystrophy • Myopathy • Muscle weakness

Chronic muscle weakness is a common complaint among patients seen in rheumatology and neuromuscular specialty clinics. This article focuses on adult-onset muscular dystrophies, select hereditary myopathies, and other neuromuscular conditions that must be distinguished from acquired causes of inflammatory muscle disease such as polymyositis. A few organizing principles help to focus the evaluation and narrow the differential diagnosis.

Because the onset of muscle weakness is typically quite insidious in genetically mediated conditions, the history provided by the patient may not at first fully reflect the degree and duration of muscle dysfunction. Individuals with long-standing and slowly progressive weakness are often able to make remarkable adaptations that permit them to function at home and in the workplace. These patients may not seek medical attention until some critical day-to-day function is finally severely impaired or lost. Because of this, it is important to question patients about physical performance and activity in relation to peers in childhood and adolescence, participation in organized sports or other physically demanding hobbies, and any physical accommodations that may have become necessary over time. These key areas of inquiry often establish a time course of disease that is much longer than initially reported. Family history may provide further diagnostic assistance; however, early parental death, variable penetrance of some diseases, recessive inheritance, de novo mutations, and other factors may obscure the genetic basis of a patient's disorder. For this reason, even in the absence of family history, the possibility of a muscular dystrophy or other genetically mediated myopathy should be considered in any adult with chronic progressive muscle weakness.

The physical examination helps to eliminate other possible neurologic disorders. The appearance of the muscles and pattern of weakness is important. A proximal and symmetric distribution of weakness is most common. With a few notable

The author has nothing to disclose.

Electromyography Laboratory, Department of Neurology, University of Colorado Denver, Academic office 1 – MS B-185, 12631 East 17th Avenue, Room 5121, Aurora, CO 80045, USA

E-mail address: Dianna.quan@ucdenver.edu

Rheum Dis Clin N Am 37 (2011) 233–244

doi:10.1016/j.rdc.2011.01.006

0889-857X/11/$ – see front matter © 2011 Elsevier Inc. All rights reserved.

rheumatic.theclinics.com

exceptions discussed herein, marked asymmetry is uncommon in dystrophies and other hereditary myopathies, and should prompt consideration of central nervous system or peripheral nerve disorders. Other patterns, such as cranial or bulbar weakness and predominantly distal extremity weakness, can occasionally be observed. Prominent fasciculations or increased muscle tone are also unusual in hereditary muscle disease and suggest anterior horn cell or central nervous system disorders, respectively. Reflexes should be normal in myopathies or may be hypoactive if muscles are severely weak. Sensation should be normal, and the presence of objective sensory disturbances indicates that weakness is most likely related to peripheral nerve or central nervous system dysfunction.

DIAGNOSTIC EVALUATION

Once a patient is determined to have neuromuscular weakness without sensory loss, the first step is to classify the process as originating in muscle, neuromuscular junction, or motor nerves or neurons. An elevated serum creatine phosphokinase (CPK) level is common in muscle disease, but milder elevations may also be observed with muscle loss from anterior horn cell or motor nerve damage. A normal CPK value does not exclude underlying muscle disease. Neuromuscular junction disease such as myasthenia gravis and Lambert-Eaton myasthenic syndrome does not affect CPK levels, but tests for acetylcholine receptor or voltage-gated P/Q calcium channel antibodies, respectively, are quite specific. In situations where blood work is not helpful, detailed high-quality electrodiagnostic testing is another important method of differentiating among the possibilities.

Patients who have unequivocal elevations in CPK levels, for example, several thousand units per liter, require further testing for muscle disease. For individuals who manifest a clear phenotype and familial pattern, genetic testing can be performed through any of several commercial or university based laboratories listed on the www.genetests.org Web site, sponsored jointly by the National Center for Biotechnology Information, the National Institutes of Health, and the University of Washington, Seattle. In patients who have no family history or distinguishing clinical features, biopsy of a weak muscle allows for routine and specialized immunohistochemical analysis that can guide more targeted genetic testing. An adequate sample is critical, whether obtained through an open procedure or needle biopsy. The choice of muscle for biopsy is also important. A strong muscle or a severely weak muscle are both less likely to be informative than a muscle that is moderately weak. It is also important to avoid a muscle that was recently examined with needle electromyography, as localized and transient inflammation may occur, causing diagnostic confusion.

The remainder of this article considers a diagnostic approach for adults with chronic progressive muscle weakness, and discusses specific muscular dystrophies and genetically mediated myopathies with 3 main patterns of clinical presentation: limb girdle weakness, bulbar or cranial weakness, and distal weakness. Features that may help to differentiate among the more common adult-onset muscular dystrophies and genetically mediated myopathies are reviewed. Disease-specific treatments and supportive therapies are discussed.

CLINICAL SYNDROMES
Limb Girdle Weakness

Dystrophinopathies
X-linked dystrophinopathies including Duchenne (DMD) and Becker (BMD) muscular dystrophy are the most common cause of muscular dystrophy. Patients with classic

DMD and BMD present with symmetric proximal muscle weakness in infancy and childhood, and are usually easily identified. In adults, the spectrum of dystrophin-related diseases may be more subtle, and is increasingly understood to be broader than originally recognized. Female carriers of dystrophin mutations may have mild muscle weakness and early cardiomyopathy. Dilated cardiomyoapthy may sometimes be the only manifestation of dystrophin abnormalities.[1] Rarely, young men with dystrophin mutations may present with exertional rhabdomyolysis and cramps without weakness between episodes.[2]

Limb girdle muscular dystrophy

Before the advent of genetic testing, patients with dystrophic muscle weakness who did not meet criteria for DMD, BMD, or other recognized syndromes were classified as limb girdle muscular dystrophy (LGMD). Clinically, patients describe weakness that mainly affects muscles in the shoulder and hip girdles. In recent decades, advances in our understanding of muscle protein structure and genetics have revealed LGMD to be a heterogeneous group of disorders with both autosomal dominant and recessive inheritance. Current classification relies on an alpha-numeric scheme. Type 1 syndromes are dominant and type 2 are recessive. The list of subtypes, grouped according to the implicated protein, is ever-expanding.[3,4]

Among the dominant mutations, defects of myotilin, lamin A/C, and caveolin-3 are the best described: LGMD 1A, LGMD 1B, and LGMD 1C, respectively. Other dominant subtypes await further characterization. The known recessive mutations are more numerous and involve alterations in γ, α, β, and δ components of the sarcoglycan complex, as well as other muscle-related proteins. Among some populations, up to 50% of patients may have no identifiable known defect.[5] Although all LGMD patients have proximal muscle weakness involving the shoulder and pelvic girdles, distinct phenotypic or clinical characteristics are recognized (**Table 1**). With standard histologic techniques, biopsy specimens demonstrate variation in fiber size, increased numbers of central nuclei, and endomysial fibrosis, changes that are common to all

Table 1
Clinical features of select limb girdle muscular dystrophies (LGMD)

LGMD Type	Gene Product	Onset (Years)	CPK (× ULN)	Special Features
Dominant				
LGMD 1A	Myotilin	>20	<5	Dysarthria; muscle inflammation; rimmed vacuoles
LGMD 1B	Lamin A/C	<20	<5	Spinal rigidity
LGMD 1C	Caveolin-3	Any	>5	—
Recessive				
LGMD 2A	Calpain-3	<40	>5	Focal muscle atrophy
LGMD 2B	Dysferlin	10–40	>10	Muscle inflammation
LGMD 2C–F	Sarcoglycan	<20	>5	Macroglossia
LGMD 2G	Telethonin	10–30	2–20	Brazilian patients; rimmed vacuoles
LGMD 2I	FKRP	Any	>5	Macroglossia
LGMD 2J	Titin	>30	<5	Rimmed vacuoles

Abbreviations: CPK, creatine phosphokinase; FKRP, Fukutin-related protein; ULN, upper limit of normal.

dystrophic muscle. In some LGMD subtypes, a few features may create confusion and suggest acquired myositis. In particular, LGMD 1A (myotilin) and LGMD 2B (dysferlin) may demonstrate inflammatory infiltrates, whereas LGMD 1A, LGMD 2G (telethonin), and LGMD 2J (titin) may have rimmed vacuoles reminiscent of inclusion body myositis.

Myotonic muscular dystrophy

Among the other muscular dystrophies that cause a limb girdle pattern of weakness, myotonic muscular dystrophy (MMD) has the unique feature of myotonia, characterized by complaints of difficulty relaxing after muscle contraction. Grip or percussion myotonia can often be elicited on physical examination. Types 1 and 2 are recognized. Type 2 is more easily confused with other LGMDs because of the more proximal distribution of weakness, whereas type 1 patients may initially complain more of hand weakness. Both are autosomal dominant with varying degrees of clinical involvement within members of the same family. Type 1 is associated with a CTG repeat expansion in the dystrophia myotonica protein kinase (DMPK) gene that encodes a serine/threonine protein kinase. Type 2 has a CCTG repeat expansion of the zinc finger protein 9 (ZNF9), encoding nucleic acid binding protein. In both conditions, the resulting expanded RNA forms nuclear inclusions in muscle cells.[6] Electrodiagnostic testing of affected muscles usually reveals characteristic myotonic discharges, and genetic analysis of blood is commercially available. Muscle biopsy is usually unnecessary due to the characteristic phenotype, electrophysiology, and ease of genetic testing. A wide range of complaints and disability exists among patients with both types of MMD, although individuals with type 1 are more often adversely affected than those with type 2. Cardiac conduction disturbances, impaired cognition, endocrine abnormalities, and early cataracts are some of the more common associated findings.

Fascioscapulohumeral muscular dystrophy

Fascioscapulohumeral muscular dystrophy (FSHD) is a relatively common autosomal dominant muscular dystrophy with a distinct distribution of weakness, usually beginning in the face and shoulder girdle and progressing into the legs over time.[7] Facial weakness is generally not debilitating, but most affected individuals are unable to whistle or may have trouble drinking from a straw. Scapular winging and difficulty raising the arms overhead are common early findings. Eventually, weakness in the lower legs becomes noticeable and progresses toward the hip girdle. Complaints of muscle fatigue and pain overlap with many rheumatologic conditions. Disease severity and progression is variable within families. Infants and children may be symptomatic, but some mildly affected individuals may not come to medical attention until well into adulthood, if at all, making the hereditary aspect of the disorder difficult to establish in some cases. New mutations and mosaicism may further obscure the genetic basis of symptoms. Most patients have a deletion of the D4Z4 tandem repeat at 4q35, but the mechanism of its deleterious effect is uncertain. Unlike the other muscular dystrophies previously discussed, FSHD often has an asymmetric distribution, especially at onset. Extramuscular manifestations are generally mild but may include retinal telangiectasias and, rarely, retinal exudation and detachment (Coat syndrome), high-frequency hearing loss, and occasional atrial arrhythmias.

Nondystrophic myopathies

Nondystrophic myopathies are relatively uncommon causes of adult-onset limb girdle weakness. The mechanisms of these disorders are varied and relate to problems such as underlying enzymatic deficiencies, collagen defects, or thin filament abnormalities.

Numerous recent monographs provide excellent reviews.[8,9] Two representative disorders warrant further discussion, due to the availability of disease-specific therapy.

Acid α-glucosidase deficiency, also known as Pompe disease, is a rare autosomal recessive condition related to abnormal degradation of lysosomal glycogen. Infants who have complete or nearly complete enzyme deficiency develop severe weakness and multisystem organ failure. In late-onset patients who have more residual enzyme activity, a progressive limb girdle pattern of weakness results. Respiratory weakness may be early and prominent. Electrodiagnostic testing shows chronic myopathic changes. Abnormalities of muscle histology in adult-onset cases may be subtle, but careful examination reveals intracytoplasmic vacuoles that stain positively with acid phosphatase. Sequence analysis of DNA from blood and enzymatic analysis of muscle are commercially available. Small studies suggest that α-glucosidase enzymatic replacement therapy may be beneficial for affected individuals.[10,11]

Among lipid storage disorders, the myopathic variant of primary carnitine deficiency may present in young adults with complaints of proximal weakness and exercise intolerance with or without myalgia. The disease is autosomal recessive and related to defective activity of the OCTN2 carnitine transporter encoded on chromosome 5. Electrodiagnostic testing shows myopathic changes, and muscle biopsy demonstrates accumulation of lipid droplets within muscle fibers. Free and total carnitine levels confirm a deficiency. Oral carnitine supplementation and reduction of dietary long-chain fatty acids with substitution of a medium-chain triglyceride diet may reduce symptoms in some patients.[12]

Nonmuscular disorders

In addition to the muscle disorders described, several other neurological conditions may superficially resemble myopathies with a limb girdle pattern of weakness. The most important to consider are disorders of motor neurons and neuromuscular junction diseases. Degeneration of lower motor neurons or anterior horn cells in the spinal cord may result in a syndrome of limb girdle weakness. In adults, the mechanisms of disease are variable. Some cases may be autosomal recessive and linked to survival motor neuron (SMN4) gene deletions or point mutations, the same locus affected in infantile and childhood forms of spinal muscular atrophy. Other cases, referred to as progressive muscular atrophy, are more often sporadic and may sometimes be early presentations of amyotrophic lateral sclerosis. Electrodiagnostic testing differentiates these neuronopathies from myopathic disorders.

In the case of neuromuscular junction disorders, the clinical features of myasthenia gravis are generally easily distinguished from myopathic limb girdle syndromes, although some diagnostic confusion may arise between myasthenia gravis and muscle disorders with prominent bulbar or cranial involvement. By contrast, Lambert-Eaton myasthenic syndrome can initially be confused for a limb girdle myopathy because of its pattern of insidious proximal muscle weakness. However, most patients have antibodies to presynaptic voltage-gated P/Q calcium channel antibodies, which are quite specific for the disorder. Electrodiagnostic testing with repetitive stimulation may be helpful, but this technique may not be performed routinely in laboratories that are less familiar with neuromuscular conditions. While about 40% of cases are autoimmune rather than paraneoplastic, a detailed search for cancer, especially small cell lung cancer, is essential in any antibody-positive patient. Treatment is directed toward eradicating the underlying neoplasm, if any. Symptomatic improvement has been reported using intravenous gammaglobulin and 3,4-diaminopuridine, which currently must be obtained and administered with approval from the Food and Drug Administration under site-specific investigational new drug applications.[13]

Craniobulbar Weakness

Oculopharyngeal muscular dystrophy

In older adults with prominent bulbar weakness, one consideration is oculopharyngeal muscular dystrophy (OPMD). This disorder was originally described among French Canadians but is known to have a worldwide distribution.[14] Symptoms begin in the fifth or sixth decade with ptosis and progressive limitation of eye movements. As is the case for other myopathies with external ophthalmoplegia, diplopia is rare. Swallowing difficulties commonly develop, increasing the risk of aspiration. Most patients exhibit mild proximal limb weakness. The disease is autosomal dominant, but due to the relatively late onset and variability of symptom severity, the familial pattern may be difficult to appreciate without detailed questioning or examination of family members. Genetic testing for a polyalanine GCG repeat expansion or unique exon duplication in the PABP gene on chromosome 14 confirms the diagnosis.

Other muscular dystrophies

Two of the previously mentioned diseases, FSHD and MMD type 1, are both associated with notable facial weakness in addition to prominent limb weakness. Patients with myotonic dystrophy commonly have ptosis, limitation of ocular motility, and temporal wasting. Mitochondrial myopathies are another consideration in patients with cranial weakness, especially those with ptosis and progressive external ophthalmoplegia.

Nonmuscular disorders

Spinal and bulbar muscular atrophy (Kennedy disease) may give the appearance of a cranial myopathy, but belongs in the category of neurogenic diseases. Adult males develop dysphagia, dysarthria, facial weakness, and mild limb weakness, beginning in the fourth and fifth decades. The disease is X-linked and associated with a CAG trinucleotide repeat on the androgen receptor gene. Prominent perioral and tongue fasciculations distinguish the disorder from myopathies. Gynecomastia and impotence are also common. Electrodiagnostic testing reveals the disease's neurogenic origin, and genetic testing provides confirmation.

Similarly, myasthenia gravis usually has prominent and early bulbar weakness. However, diurnal fluctuation of symptoms and frequent diplopia distinguish it clinically from other primary muscle disorders. Electrophysiologic evaluation and serum antibody testing are key steps in diagnosis. Early recognition is important, because progression to life-threatening respiratory weakness and dysphagia can be rapid yet fully reversible with treatment.

Distal Myopathies

Welander and Udd distal myopathy

Not all primary muscle disease results in proximal symmetric weakness. Distally predominant myopathies are relatively uncommon in American adults but warrant consideration in patients who complain of distal weakness without sensory disturbances. Different types are endemic to various parts of the globe. Individuals of Scandinavian descent are most often affected by the Welander form, with prevalence in Sweden being as high as 1 in 1000.[15] Affected patients develop hand weakness after the fourth decade followed later by leg weakness. By contrast, Udd myopathy seen in Finland manifests as weakness in the anterior compartment of the forelegs and generally does not progress to the upper extremities. Both Welander and Udd are autosomal dominant and may show rimmed vacuoles on muscle pathology, resulting in potential confusion with inclusion body myositis.

Miyoshi myopathy

In Japan, China, and other parts of the world, Miyoshi distal myopathy is more common. Symptoms begin in adolescence to mid adulthood and are characterized by lower leg involvement. Initially problems may be limited to myalgia and exercise intolerance, especially after physical activity, and the calf muscles may be bulky. As the disease progresses, most patients experience weakness in the calf muscles first, but occasional patients may develop early foot drop. Over time patients may lose the ability to walk. In the early stages, CPK is often strikingly high. The disease is autosomal recessive and is allelic with LGMD 2B. Histologically, inflammation and vacuoles may be seen, suggesting acquired polymyositis or inclusion body myositis, but immunostaining reveals a characteristic deficiency of dysferlin. Within the same family, phenotypic variability is common.

Nonaka myopathy

Another distal myopathy with rimmed vacuoles has been described among patients from many parts of the world, with larger affected populations in the Middle East and Japan. Bilateral foot drop in adolescence or early to mid adulthood eventually progresses to calf muscle weakness and proximal leg weakness. Some patients may also have inflammatory changes on muscle biopsy. However, unlike acquired inclusion body myositis, there is relative sparing of the quadriceps muscles. DNA sequence analysis and targeted mutation analysis are available in laboratories around the world.

Other adult-onset distal myopathies

A few other muscle disorders may present with predominant distal weakness; these include myofibrillary myopathy, multi-minicore disease, and nemaline myopathy. While relatively uncommon, the characteristic findings on muscle biopsy in each of these disorders are revealing: large nonrimmed vacuoles and focal subsarcolemmal or intrasarcoplasmic masses in myofibrillar myopathy, and multi-minicores and nemaline rods in the eponymous myopathies. Other considerations in the setting of distal weakness include dystrophies such as MMD type 1 where complaints of hand weakness may be prominent, or FSHD and LGMD 2J where complaints of lower leg weakness may be prominent.

Other Patterns and Distinguishing Features

The preceding discussion, based on 3 major clinical patterns of muscle weakness, provides a general overview of more common dystrophic and nondystrophic genetic myopathies. Distinctive systemic features may further aid in the recognition of specific disorders. A few important associations including cardiac disease, muscle hypertrophy, joint hypermobility, joint contractures, and respiratory weakness have been chosen for discussion here.

Cardiac involvement

Cardiac muscle can be adversely affected in many muscular dystrophies. In some patients these abnormalities remain relatively asymptomatic, and limitations in physical activity due to limb weakness further mask symptoms. Individuals with typical DMD and BMD fall into this group. In other patients, cardiac manifestations predominate over those of skeletal muscle. This situation may be seen in patients with Danon disease, who have an X-linked dominant defect of lysosomal associated membrane protein 2 (LAMP 2) and a vacuolar myopathy. Affected individuals may have mild or no limb girdle weakness, but have conduction defects or cardiomyopathy so severe that pacemakers or heart transplantation become necessary.[16] In yet other patients, such as those with MMD, the cardiac and skeletal muscle disease are equally important. **Table 2** summarizes important associations between cardiac and muscle disease.

Muscle hypertrophy
Enlargement of muscles can occur early in the course of many muscle conditions. Calf hypertrophy can be a helpful clinical finding and may be seen in dystrophinopathies, some LGMD variants, especially sarcoglycan disorders, MMD type 2, and late-onset Pompe disease. Enlarged calf muscles may also be observed in patients with myotonia congenita, most of whom carry a mutation in the CLCN1 gene regulating chloride channel function. Patients with myotonia congenita typically complain less of true muscle weakness and more of difficulties relaxing muscle or moving muscles after a period of rest.

Joint hypermobility and contractures
Abnormalities of joint mobility have been associated with several muscle disorders in adults. Examples include LGMD 2A, Bethlem myopathy, multi-minicore myopathy, and central core myopathy. Some individuals with Bethlem myopathy may not be aware of significant weakness but may note flexion contractures of the fingers, wrists, elbows, and ankles. Hypermobility of distal interphalangeal joints can coexist with contractures. Weakness usually progresses slowly, although over decades patients may lose the ability to walk. In multi-minicore disease, contractures are common but may be as subtle and limited as Achilles tendon tightness. Concomitant joint hypermobility is observed in the hands, and patellar and knee dislocations may occur

Table 2
Summary of select clinical features

Condition	Cardiac	Respiratory	Hypertrophy	Contractures	Hypermobility	Scapular Winging	Other
LGMD 1B	CM	+	—	+	—	—	—
LGMD 2A	—	—	—	+	—	+	—
LGMD 2C	CM	+	+	—	—	+	—
LGMD 2D	+/−	+	+	—	—	+	—
LGMD 2E	CM	+	+	+	+	+	—
LGMD 2F	CM	+	+	—	—	—	—
LGMD 2I	CM	+	+	—	—	—	—
MMD type 1	CD	—	—	—	—	—	—
MMD type 2	+/−	—	+	—	—	—	—
FSHD	—	—	—	—	—	+	—
Danon	CM/CD	—	—	—	—	—	—
Pompe	CM	+	+	—	—	—	—
Nemaline	CM	—	—	—	—	—	MH
Myofibrillar	CM	—	—	—	—	—	—
Bethlem	—	+	—	+	+	—	—
MMC	—	+	—	+	+	—	MH
Central core	—	—	—	—	+	—	MH

Abbreviations: CD, conduction defects; CM, cardiomyopathy; MH, susceptibility to malignant hyperthermia with ryanodine receptor 1 associated disease; MMC, multi-minicore.

due to ligamentous laxity. Weakness mostly affects axial muscles and is usually slowly progressive. Similarly, central core myopathy is also associated with axial muscle and hip girdle weakness with ligamentous laxity and joint hypermobility. Widespread contractures are uncommon. Genetic testing is available for all of these disorders.

Respiratory muscle weakness
Respiratory weakness in the setting of Pompe disease has already been mentioned. Other adult-onset muscle disorders, including LGMD 1B, sarcoglycan LGMDs, LGMD 2I, Bethlem myopathy, and multi-minicore myopathy, may also have prominent and early respiratory weakness. While the breathing impairment in all of these conditions can eventually be severe, the pace of worsening develops gradually over months and years.

TREATMENT
Disease-Specific Therapies

In disorders where the genetic mutation and protein defects are known, therapeutic strategies have focused on replacing specific genes or proteins, finding mutation-specific treatments, boosting alternative proteins, and modulating other pathways that lead to muscle dysfunction. In situations where a specific protein is missing or the levels inadequate, replacement of the protein or gene that encodes it is the most obvious conceptual approach. This approach has become possible in disorders such as Pompe disease, where enzyme replacement therapy has become a commercial reality. The replacement of a gene encoding cellular structural components is more problematic in that a targeted delivery system, and in the case of viral vectors the development of appropriate immune modulation, must first be achieved.

In some cases, the size of the genetic defect or size and complexity of the encoded protein prohibit a direct replacement approach, and mutation specific techniques may allow more fruitful therapies. Efforts in this regard have focused on the most common dystrophin disorder DMD, where a frame shift in the DNA reading frame results from a large deletion. Use of antisense oligonucleotides to modify messenger RNA and restore the reading frame have led to promising preclinical studies in DMD as well as other DNA expansion disorders such as MMD.[17,18]

Where compensatory mechanisms are known to exist, strategies to boost these pathways have provided another avenue for ameliorating muscle disease. Attempts to upregulate utrophin expression in DMD are an example of this.[19] Other potential targets for this type of gene therapy have been identified in some congenital muscular dystrophies, MMD type 1, and various forms of LGMD. Consideration of direct administration of a compensatory protein is also under consideration as in the case of lamin-111, which improves the dystrophic phenotype in a mouse model of muscular dystrophy.[20] How well these approaches would be tolerated and the extent of their clinical benefits in people remains to be seen.

Beyond deficient or defective proteins, the severity and course of muscle disease is clearly modified by posttranslational factors. Strategies to decrease calcium overload, protect mitochondria, and enhance muscle growth may provide therapeutic options that are widely applicable in chronic muscle disease. However, based on clinical and pathologic observations, at least some of the mechanisms leading to muscle degeneration, necrosis, and impaired regeneration are unique to each disorder. An interesting observation in MMD type 2 reveals a possible association with autoimmune diseases.[21] In a small cohort of patients, individuals with MMD type 2 had a notably higher frequency of autoimmune disorders than MMD type 1 patients or the general population. Whether this observation relates to MMD type 2 directly influencing development of immune system changes via an RNA-mediated mechanism or whether the presence of an MMD type 2 expansion increases susceptibility to autoimmune disorders via other genetic factors requires further investigation.

Clues from histologic differences among the dystrophies have also been of interest. The prominent inflammatory changes seen in muscles of patients with dystrophinopathies or defects of dysferlin have led to speculation that progressive muscle damage in these conditions involves important immune-mediated factors that may be potential therapeutic targets. In DMD, corticosteroids have been used clinically for many years to provide transient improvement in muscle strength and function and in respiratory function. In part, the mechanism of steroid action may be anti-inflammatory or immunosuppressive.[22] However, in the dysferlin deficiency disorders Miyoshi myopathy and LGMD 2B, steroids have not had even the limited success found in DMD. Other factors are clearly operative and remain to be explored.[23,24]

Supportive Therapies

In the absence of widely available disease-specific treatments, supportive measures play an important role in maintaining function and improving quality of life. In disorders where other systemic manifestations can develop, routine monitoring is essential; this is especially true in the case of cardiopulmonary involvement. Symptomatic patients clearly require urgent and more detailed testing. In asymptomatic patients, no definite consensus exists for the exact frequency and methods of assessing cardiopulmonary status. In MDM type 1, some helpful data are available. Groh and colleagues[25] found that a clinical diagnosis of atrial tachyarrhythmia or severe electrocardiographic (ECG) abnormalities, defined as a rhythm other than sinus, PR interval of 240 milliseconds or more, QRS duration of 120 milliseconds or more, or second- or third-degree atrioventricular block, were independent risk factors for sudden death. Atrial tachyarrhythmias were seen both among patients who had severe ECG abnormalities and among those who did not, although they were more common in the former group. The study did not reveal a reduction in cardiac mortality with the use of implanted pacemakers or cardioverter-defibrillators, although addressing this question was not the primary purpose of the study. In the absence of more robust data, yearly ECG testing with formal cardiology evaluation for abnormal findings seems a reasonable method of screening asymptomatic patients with muscle disorders known to have important cardiac manifestations.

Respiratory compromise in muscle disorders is generally less of a concern in adult-onset disease than in infantile or childhood conditions. Patients may self-report shortness of breath at rest or with exertion. Routine questions regarding morning headaches, daytime fatigue or sleepiness, and poor quality of sleep also help to identify patients who may have hypercapnea during sleep. In adults, weakness of respiratory muscles that seems out of proportion to limb weakness should prompt consideration of specific conditions (see **Table 2**). Baseline testing of the forced vital capacity is a convenient and painless way to identify patients who may benefit from noninvasive positive pressure ventilatory (NPPV) support. Use of NPPV support, especially at night, improves health-related quality of life and extends life in many neuromuscular conditions, although specific data on most adult-onset muscular dystrophies and myopathies are lacking.[26,27]

Common to all dystrophies and myopathies are physical impairments that may limit gait or upper extremity function and other day-to-day activities. Options to support mobility range from canes or walkers, to increasingly lightweight and flexible orthotic devices, to sophisticated power chairs. For the arms and hands, simple adaptive mechanical devices may help preserve independent activities such as eating and dressing. Deterioration in handwriting can be overcome with the aid of computer and voice recognition technology. For patients with dysphagia, nutritional supplementation may become necessary, and if weight loss becomes progressive, percutaneous gastrostomy tube feeding should be considered. The loss of independence occasioned by these limitations may have profound emotional and psychological consequences that should not be ignored. Family and social structures should be supported where possible, and patients should be encouraged to remain as active as possible in their homes and communities. When necessary, formal counseling or medication for depression and anxiety should be prescribed.

SUMMARY

A wide variety of neuromuscular conditions may present with progressive weakness. The differential diagnosis of adult-onset myopathies should encompass muscular dystrophies and genetically mediated myopathies. Other conditions should be considered depending on the distribution of weakness, electrodiagnostic findings, associated clinical features, and muscle histology and immunohistochemistry. Although current disease-specific treatments lag behind our knowledge of the affected genes and proteins for many muscle disorders, continuing scientific advances offer a promising future. In the interim, improvements in supportive therapies allow affected individuals to maintain a meaningful quality of life.

REFERENCES

1. Cohen N, Muntoni F. Multiple pathogenetic mechanisms in X linked dilated cardiomyopathy. Heart 2004;90:835–41.
2. Figarella-Branger D, Baeta Machado AM, Putzu GA, et al. Exertional rhabdomyolysis and exercise intolerance revealing dystrophinopathies. Acta Neuropathol 1997;94:48–53.
3. Norwood F, de Visser M, Eymard B, et al. EFNS guideline on diagnosis and management of limb girdle muscular dystrophies. Eur J Neurol 2007;14:1305–12.
4. Guglieri M, Straub V, Bushby K, et al. Limb-girdle muscular dystrophies. Curr Opin Neurol 2008;21:576–84.
5. Sunada Y. Limb-girdle muscular dystrophy; update. Rinsho Shinkeigaku 2004;44:995–7 [in Japanese].
6. Wheeler TM, Thornton CA. Myotonic dystrophy: RNA-mediated muscle disease. Curr Opin Neurol 2007;20:572–6.
7. Padberg GW, van Engelen BG. Facioscapulohumeral muscular dystrophy. Curr Opin Neurol 2009;22:539–42.
8. Sewry CA, Jimenez-Mallebrera C, Muntoni F. Congenital myopathies. Curr Opin Neurol 2008;21:569–75.
9. Sharma MC, Jain D, Sarkar C, et al. Congenital myopathies—a comprehensive update of recent advancements. Acta Neurol Scand 2009;119:281–92.
10. Ravaglia S, Danesino C, Moglia A, et al. Changes in nutritional status and body composition during enzyme replacement therapy in adult-onset type II glycogenosis. Eur J Neurol 2010;17(7):957–62.
11. Wokke JH, Escolar DM, Pestronk A, et al. Clinical features of late-onset Pompe disease: a prospective cohort study. Muscle Nerve 2008;38:1236–45.
12. Vielhaber S, Feistner H, Weis J, et al. Primary carnitine deficiency: adult onset lipid storage myopathy with a mild clinical course. J Clin Neurosci 2004;11:919–24.

13. Maddison P, Newsom-Davis J. Treatment for Lambert-Eaton myasthenic syndrome. Cochrane Database Syst Rev 2005;2:CD003279.
14. Abu-Baker A, Rouleau GA. Oculopharyngeal muscular dystrophy: recent advances in the understanding of the molecular pathogenic mechanisms and treatment strategies. Biochim Biophys Acta 2007;1772:173–85.
15. Udd B, Bushby K, Nonaka I, et al. 104th European Neuromuscular Centre (ENMC) International Workshop: distal myopathies, 8–10th March 2002 in Naarden, The Netherlands. Neuromuscul Disord 2002;12:897–904.
16. Sugie K, Yamamoto A, Murayama K, et al. Clinicopathological features of genetically confirmed Danon disease. Neurology 2002;58:1773–8.
17. Aartsma-Rus A, van Ommen GJ. Progress in therapeutic antisense applications for neuromuscular disorders. Eur J Hum Genet 2010;18:146–53.
18. Wheeler TM, Sobczak K, Lueck JD, et al. Reversal of RNA dominance by displacement of protein sequestered on triplet repeat RNA. Science 2009;325: 336–9.
19. Miura P, Jasmin BJ. Utrophin upregulation for treating Duchenne or Becker muscular dystrophy: how close are we? Trends Mol Med 2006;12:122–9.
20. Rooney JE, Gurpur PB, Burkin DJ. Laminin-111 protein therapy prevents muscle disease in the mdx mouse model for Duchenne muscular dystrophy. Proc Natl Acad Sci U S A 2009;106:7991–6.
21. Tieleman AA, den Broeder AA, van de Logt AE, et al. Strong association between myotonic dystrophy type 2 and autoimmune diseases. J Neurol Neurosurg Psychiatry 2009;80:1293–5.
22. Kissel JT, Burrow KL, Rammohan KW, et al. Mononuclear cell analysis of muscle biopsies in prednisone-treated and untreated Duchenne muscular dystrophy. CIDD Study Group. Neurology 1991;41:667–72.
23. Manzur AY, Kuntzer T, Pike M, et al. Glucocorticoid corticosteroids for Duchenne muscular dystrophy. Cochrane Database Syst Rev 2008;1:CD003725.
24. Tidball JG, Wehling-Henricks M. Damage and inflammation in muscular dystrophy: potential implications and relationships with autoimmune myositis. Curr Opin Rheumatol 2005;17:707–13.
25. Groh WJ, Groh MR, Saha C, et al. Electrocardiographic abnormalities and sudden death in myotonic dystrophy type 1. N Engl J Med 2008;358:2688–97.
26. Bourke SC, Tomlinson M, Williams TL, et al. Effects of non-invasive ventilation on survival and quality of life in patients with amyotrophic lateral sclerosis: a randomised controlled trial. Lancet Neurol 2006;5:140–7.
27. Dreher M, Rauter I, Storre JH, et al. When should home mechanical ventilation be started in patients with different neuromuscular disorders? Respirology 2007;12: 749–53.

Imaging of Skeletal Muscle

Douglas W. Goodwin, MD

KEYWORDS

• Skeletal muscle • MRI • Imaging • Myositis

A variety of diagnostic imaging techniques have made possible the noninvasive evaluation of skeletal muscle injury and disease. Sonography allows for the dynamic assessment of musculotendinous structures and tissue vascularity and is particularly useful in determining whether lesions are cystic or solid.[1] Although inexpensive and widely available, the use of this technique is limited by operator experience, difficulty in imaging deep structures, a restricted field of view, and limited contrast resolution. Computed tomography acquires cross-sectional images that are valuable in imaging tissues deep in the surface that are not well displayed on routine radiographs. The technique, however, is limited by poor soft tissue contrast and the risk of radiation exposure. Radiography remains a relatively inexpensive and widely available technique for identifying calcified abnormalities such as phleboliths and heterotopic ossification. Scintigraphy is of some use in the evaluation of skeletal muscle disorders, but it lacks specificity.

Although all these different modalities have roles to play, magnetic resonance imaging (MRI) is especially sensitive in the diagnosis of muscle disorders and injury and has proved to be useful in determining the extent of disease, in directing interventions, and in monitoring the response to therapies. At the most basic level, MRI creates images by exploiting the predictable behavior of protons placed in a strong magnetic field. The images largely reflect the distribution of protons within fat and water. The signal intensity of any tissue is therefore largely a reflection of the proton density of a particular tissue. However, the behavior of protons in these tissues is strongly influenced by tissue structure and the behavior of nearby protons, and this behavior of protons influences the magnetic resonance (MR) image. T1 and T2 are constants that describe 2 behaviors of the protons of a given tissue in a magnetic field. The signal intensity of any tissue on an MR image can be altered by changing the manner in which it is created through the use of different imaging sequences. This alteration allows MR to create tissue contrast by exploiting differences in tissue composition and structure. Sequences that are T1 or T2 weighted are designed to emphasize the differences in T1 or T2, respectively.

The author has nothing to disclose.
Department of Radiology, Dartmouth-Hitchcock Medical Center, Dartmouth Medical School, One Medical Center Drive, Lebanon, NH 03756, USA
E-mail address: douglas.goodwin@hitchcock.org

doi:10.1016/j.rdc.2011.01.007
0889-857X/11/$ – see front matter
rheumatic.theclinics.com
© 2011 Elsevier Inc. All rights reserved.

On T1-weighted images, high–signal intensity adipose tissue can be seen surrounding intermediate–signal intensity skeletal muscle. These images are particularly useful for the evaluation of muscle size and the presence of anomalous muscles. Methemoglobin deposition secondary to intramuscular hematoma or a hemorrhagic neoplasm is also associated with increased signal intensity. In the setting of muscle atrophy caused by injury, inflammation, or denervation, T1-weighted images are of great value in assessing the presence and amount of intramuscular fat.[2] Gadolinium-based intravascular contrast agents can be used in conjunction with fat-suppressed T1-weighted images (**Fig. 1**). Although the value of contrast in skeletal muscle imaging is limited, it may be helpful in identifying areas of necrosis or abscess formation.

T2-weighted images are sensitive to the presence of water, which is displayed as high signal intensity. The finding of water signal, however, is not specific and may represent muscle exertion, inflammation, infection, subacute denervation, ischemia, myonecrosis, injury, or infiltrating neoplasm.[2] Although fat signal intensity is low on classic conventional spin echo images, it remains high on the newer fast spin echo T2-weighted images, which have largely replaced spin echo imaging because of the decreased scanning time required (**Fig. 2**). In order to produce truly fluid-sensitive images, it is therefore necessary to suppress the fat signal. Frequently, a saturation pulse is used to suppress the signal from protons with the frequency of fat. This fat saturation technique is routinely used with little difficulty. However, when imaging large fields of view, as is frequently the case when imaging skeletal muscle, suppression may fail at the margins of the image. This failure is the result of the diminished homogeneity of the magnetic field and associated variations in fat frequency. Frequency-selective fat suppression is also unreliable when imaging with low-field scanners.[3] In these settings, inversion recovery (IR) fast spin-spin echo imaging, an updated version of short tau IR imaging (STIR) provides reliably uniform fat suppression.

When evaluating patients with suspected myositis, the authors acquire T1-weighted and IR images in the axial plane and supplement those images with coronal plane IR

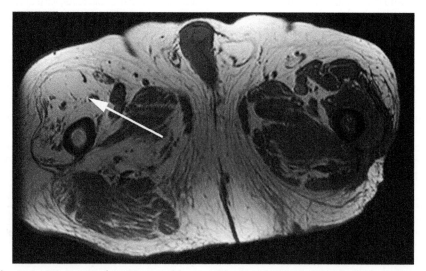

Fig. 1. An MR image of an 80-year-old man with extensive muscular atrophy secondary to polio. The T1-weighted axial image of the pelvis reveals intramuscular high–signal intensity fat, with most pronounced involvement in the right quadriceps muscles (*arrow*).

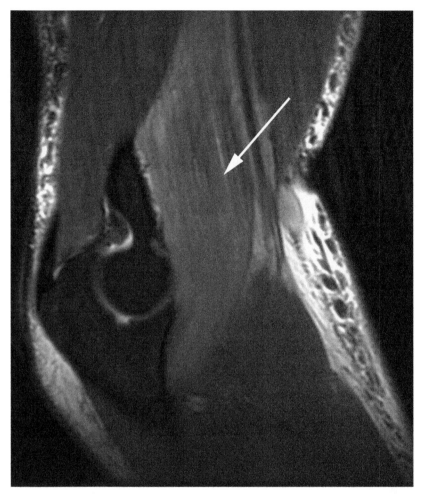

Fig. 2. MR images of a 19-year-old man with injury caused by overexertion after prolonged weightlifting. High signal intensity within the brachialis muscle (*arrow*) on this fat-saturated T2-weighted sagittal image of the elbow is a nonspecific indication of injury to muscle.

images. This protocol requires the acquisition of images at the thighs, followed by a change in the positioning of the patient and then a repeat imaging at the lower part of the legs. On some newer MR scanners, the entire body can be imaged without a change in position, allowing for the relatively rapid study of the total body. When infectious myositis is suspected, the use of gadolinium-based contrast may be useful in identifying abscesses.

Although the MRI findings of muscle inflammation are not specific, characteristic patterns of disease and injury have been described. For example, in the setting of suspected idiopathic inflammatory myopathy, little distinguishes polymyositis from dermatomyositis, but inclusion body myositis may affect the upper extremities more frequently and present with asymmetric distribution and distal involvement.[4,5] MRI may be used to establish an early diagnosis, determine disease activity and extent, assess response to therapy, and direct biopsy. In the setting of active myositis, a high signal on T2-weighted images, often referred to as muscle edema reflects the accumulation of extracellular water and inflammatory infiltrate.[6–8] In the chronic stage, muscle girth is decreased and replaced by adipose, which is well displayed on T1-weighted images.[9] By combining fluid-sensitive images, such as IR images, with T1-weighted images, both the level of active disease and the extent of chronic disease can be evaluated. MR images can be used to identify areas of active inflammation, seen as high–signal intensity areas on fluid-sensitive sequences, and minimal atrophy (**Fig. 3**). The findings of pyomyositis are similar to those of idiopathic disease, even though involvement is typically more localized and muscle enlargement is common.[10] Using imaging to target the regions of concern improves the efficacy and cost-effectiveness of biopsy or, in the setting of infection, aspiration or abscess drainage.[11]

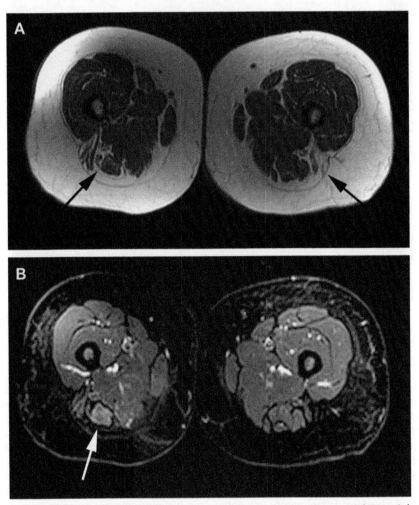

Fig. 3. MR images of a 57-year-old woman with dermatomyositis. On an axial T1-weighted image of the thighs (*A*), the presence of fat infiltration within the biceps femoris muscle bilaterally (*arrows*) indicates chronic disease and muscular atrophy. On an IR image (*B*), the high signal intensity (*arrow*) within the right biceps femoris indicates acute inflammation and the optimal location for biopsy.

In the presence of ischemia and necrosis of muscle, increased muscle size and increased signal intensity within the muscle and the surrounding fascia as displayed on T2-weighted MR images are the characteristic findings. MR is, as a result, sensitive in the diagnosis of diabetic muscle infarction, compartment syndrome, and rhabdomyolysis. When evaluating compartment syndrome, a high signal intensity on T1-weighted images indicates the presence of foci of hemorrhage. The evaluation of chronic compartment syndrome may be facilitated by imaging after a period of exercise.[12,13]

Denervation of muscle may be caused by a variety of injuries to nerve, including entrapment, trauma, inflammation, and vascular compromise.[14] MRI, often as an adjunct to electromyogram, is a powerful noninvasive diagnostic test.[15] After a nerve insult, subacute changes in muscle include the presence of high signal intensity on fluid-sensitive images with no associate abnormality on T1-weighted images.[16] Although these findings are not specific to denervation, an appropriate clinical presentation and isolation of these findings to a specific nerve territory is strongly suggestive of the diagnosis (**Fig. 4**). With chronic denervation, muscle size decreases and adipose infiltration can be seen on T1-weighted images.[17]

Trauma to muscle, including biomechanical overload, laceration, contusion, hemorrhage, and herniation, are well displayed on MR images. As with other insults to muscle, acute injury is associated with an elevation of signal intensity on fluid-sensitive sequences.[18] This finding of increased interstitial fluid may be the only imaging abnormality, as is the case with delayed-onset muscle soreness.[19] In the setting of muscle strain, focal structural distortion at the myotendinous junction accompanies the abnormal fluid signal.[20] The size of injury to the myotendinous

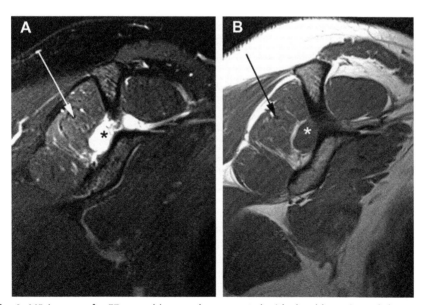

Fig. 4. MR images of a 57-year-old man who presented with shoulder pain and decreased strength. Sagittal IR (*A*) and T1-weighted (*B*) images of the shoulder reveal a paraglenoid cyst (*A, B, asterisk*). Within the infraspinatus muscle (*A, B, arrow*), the presence of high signal on both the IR and T1-weighted images is virtually diagnostic of chronic denervation caused by nerve entrapment of the infraspinatus nerve as it passes next to the spinoglenoid notch.

junction is useful in staging the injury and predicting the time needed for return to athletic activity.[21] On T1-weighted images, high signal intensity within the muscle, representing the presence of methemoglobin, indicates hemorrhage. Gradient-recalled echo imaging is particularly sensitive to the presence of calcification and can be a useful addition to routine imaging when evaluating possible heterotopic ossification or diffuse soft tissue calcification.

A variety of different MRI sequences are likely be used in the future to study skeletal muscle in greater detail. Emerging techniques include the real-time visualization of muscle contraction through the use of dynamic imaging. Functional imaging techniques such as blood oxygenation level–dependent imaging distinguish differences in tissue levels of oxyhemoglobin, and quantitative techniques such as T2 mapping can be used to investigate muscle recruitment and activation. Whereas these new techniques may well prove to be useful in the future, even the most basic applications of MRI widely available today are capable of establishing a diagnosis in a variety of skeletal muscle disorders, guiding therapeutic intervention, and monitoring the response to therapy.

REFERENCES

1. Newman JS, Adler RS, Rubin JM. Power Doppler sonography: use in measuring alterations in muscle blood volume after exercise. AJR Am J Roentgenol 1997; 168(6):1525–30.

2. Rubin DA, Kneeland JB. MR imaging of the musculoskeletal system: technical considerations for enhancing image quality and diagnostic yield. AJR Am J Roentgenol 1994;163(5):1155–63.

3. Delfaut EM, Beltran J, Johnson G, et al. Fat suppression in MR imaging: techniques and pitfalls. Radiographics 1999;19(2):373–82.

4. Dion E, Cherin P, Payan C, et al. Magnetic resonance imaging criteria for distinguishing between inclusion body myositis and polymyositis. J Rheumatol 2002; 29(9):1897–906.

5. Sekul EA, Chow C, Dalakas MC. Magnetic resonance imaging of the forearm as a diagnostic aid in patients with sporadic inclusion body myositis. Neurology 1997;48(4):863–6.

6. Garcia J. MRI in inflammatory myopathies. Skeletal Radiol 2000;29(8):425–38.

7. Hernandez RJ, Keim DR, Chenevert TL, et al. Fat-suppressed MR imaging of myositis. Radiology 1992;182(1):217–9.

8. Reimers CD, Schedel H, Fleckenstein JL, et al. Magnetic resonance imaging of skeletal muscles in idiopathic inflammatory myopathies of adults. J Neurol 1994;241(5):306–14.

9. Adams EM, Chow CK, Premkumar A, et al. The idiopathic inflammatory myopathies: spectrum of MR imaging findings. Radiographics 1995;15(3):563–74.

10. Gordon BA, Martinez S, Collins AJ. Pyomyositis: characteristics at CT and MR imaging. Radiology 1995;197(1):279–86.

11. Schweitzer ME, Fort J. Cost-effectiveness of MR imaging in evaluating polymyositis. AJR Am J Roentgenol 1995;165(6):1469–71.

12. Eskelin MK, Lotjonen JM, Mantysaari MJ. Chronic exertional compartment syndrome: MR imaging at 0.1 T compared with tissue pressure measurement. Radiology 1998;206(2):333–7.

13. Kumar PR, Jenkins JP, Hodgson SP. Bilateral chronic exertional compartment syndrome of the dorsal part of the forearm: the role of magnetic resonance imaging in diagnosis: a case report. J Bone Joint Surg Am 2003;85(8):1557–9.

14. May DA, Disler DG, Jones EA, et al. Abnormal signal intensity in skeletal muscle at MR imaging: patterns, pearls, and pitfalls. Radiographics 2000;20(Spec No): S295–315.

15. McDonald CM, Carter GT, Fritz RC, et al. Magnetic resonance imaging of denervated muscle: comparison to electromyography. Muscle Nerve 2000;23(9): 1431–4.

16. Bredella MA, Tirman PF, Fritz RC, et al. Denervation syndromes of the shoulder girdle: MR imaging with electrophysiologic correlation. Skeletal Radiol 1999; 28(10):567–72.

17. Fritz RC, Boutin RD. Magnetic resonance imaging of the peripheral nervous system. Phys Med Rehabil Clin N Am 2001;12(2):399–432.

18. El-Khoury GY, Brandser EA, Kathol MH, et al. Imaging of muscle injuries. Skeletal Radiol 1996;25(1):3–11.

19. Shellock FG, Fukunaga T, Mink JH, et al. Acute effects of exercise on MR imaging of skeletal muscle: concentric vs eccentric actions. AJR Am J Roentgenol 1991; 156(4):765–8.

20. Palmer WE, Kuong SJ, Elmadbouh HM. MR imaging of myotendinous strain. AJR Am J Roentgenol 1999;173(3):703–9.

21. Slavotinek JP, Verrall GM, Fon GT. Hamstring injury in athletes: using MR imaging measurements to compare extent of muscle injury with amount of time lost from competition. AJR Am J Roentgenol 2002;179(6):1621–8.

A Primer on Electrophysiologic Studies in Myopathy

Matthew C. Lynch, MD[a], Jeffrey A. Cohen, MD[a,b],*

KEYWORDS

• Electromyography • Myopathy • Myositis
• Neurophysiology • Neuropathic disease

PURPOSE AND LIMITATIONS

The purpose of electromyography (EMG) is to localize a lesion within the peripheral nervous system. Peripheral causes of weakness can be divided into neuropathic processes, myopathic processes, and diseases affecting the neuromuscular junction. A neuropathic process is one which affects the anterior horn cell or its axon as it passes through the nerve root, plexus, or peripheral nerve. A myopathic process affects the muscle fibers. Specialized techniques can be performed, if necessary, to evaluate the neuromuscular junction. Weakness caused by disorders of the central nervous system such as multiple sclerosis or stroke is not usually diagnosed with EMG. This review focuses on physiologic principles involved in differentiating lesions of the lower motor neuron from primary muscle diseases.

Electrodiagnostic testing has some important limitations. A few muscle diseases do not cause abnormalities on EMG. Any muscle disease affecting the contractile apparatus of muscle fibers without affecting their electrical properties would not be detectable on EMG (eg, some congenital or endocrine myopathies).[1] A normal EMG can also be seen in the setting of steroid myopathy. This condition causes atrophy preferentially of type II muscle fibers,[2–4] but EMG detects primarily type I fibers during the weaker levels of contraction at which individual motor units can be seen.[5] Thus, a normal EMG would not rule out these conditions.

Even an abnormal EMG by itself does not often produce a specific diagnosis, because there are no findings that are specific to any given disease.[1] For example, electrical myotonia is almost always observed in myotonic dystrophy, but can also be seen in other conditions such as paramyotonia congenita, acid maltase deficiency,

The authors have nothing to disclose.
a Department of Neurology, Dartmouth Hitchcock Medical Center, 1 Medical Center Drive, Lebanon, NH 03756, USA
b Department of Neurology, Dartmouth Medical School, Hanover, NH, USA
* Corresponding author. Department of Neurology, Dartmouth Hitchcock Medical Center, 1 Medical Center Drive, Lebanon, NH 03756.
E-mail address: Jeffrey.A.Cohen@hitchcock.org

Rheum Dis Clin N Am 37 (2011) 253–268
doi:10.1016/j.rdc.2011.01.008
0889-857X/11/$ – see front matter © 2011 Elsevier Inc. All rights reserved.

or rarely in neuropathic conditions. However, sometimes clinical history and examination findings supplement the electrophyisologic results to produce a specific diagnosis. Suppose EMG reveals myotonia in a 45-year-old man with weakness of the distal hand muscles, ankle dorsiflexors, and face. He also has frontal balding, cataracts, and diabetes mellitus. There is a family history of weakness in a similar pattern showing genetic anticipation. This patient can be diagnosed without further testing as having myotonic dystrophy because of the characteristic clinical history and EMG myotonia. At other times EMG aids diagnosis by localizing the pathology to muscle, directing further diagnostic testing such as muscle biopsy or genetic testing, which can be helpful in making a specific diagnosis. EMG can also be helpful in selecting an affected muscle for biopsy. Typically a biopsy site contralateral to the limb examined with EMG would be chosen, because damage from the EMG needle may affect biopsy results.[6]

PRINCIPLES OF MUSCLE PHYSIOLOGY

A brief review of basic nerve and muscle physiology serves as a foundation on which to build understanding of common EMG findings. Muscles are organized into motor units. A motor unit consists of a single alpha motor neuron and all of the muscle fibers it innervates, as shown in **Fig. 1**A. One motor neuron may innervate several muscle fibers (in muscles requiring high precision such as extraocular muscles) or hundreds of muscle fibers (in muscles requiring steady power such as the gastrocnemius). The muscle fibers of a single motor unit are not situated adjacent to each other.

When a motor neuron fires, an action potential propagates down its axon and all of the axon twigs. When the action potential reaches the nerve terminal, the depolarization triggers opening of voltage-gated calcium channels. The influx of calcium then triggers the release of acetylcholine into the extracellular space by fusion of the storage vesicles with the muscle membrane. Acetylcholine diffuses across the neuromuscular junction and activates nicotinic receptors, which are ligand-gated sodium channels. The influx of sodium into the muscle cell triggers an action potential in the muscle fiber similar to that in the nerve. However, muscle fibers contain a system of tunnels (called transverse or "T" tubules), which are invaginations of the cell membrane into the depths of the muscle cell, allowing the action potential to propagate rapidly throughout the muscle cell. The lumen of the T tubule is contiguous with the extracellular space. T tubules lie adjacent to an intracellular system of tunnels called the sarcoplasmic reticulum, which is a repository for stored calcium. The depolarization of the T tubules triggers voltage-gated calcium channels, leading to an initial calcium influx into the muscle fiber. This process causes the further release of calcium stores in the sarcoplasmic reticulum. The accumulation of calcium in the muscle fiber then drives the contractile apparatus. The flux of ions within muscle fiber creates an electric field that can be recorded from the EMG needle.

In neuropathic conditions the motor axon is injured, leaving muscle fibers of entire motor units without innervation. The muscle fibers become hyperexcitable, leading to spontaneous depolarization and contraction of a single muscle fiber, which is detected on EMG as fibrillations or positive sharp wave potentials. The denervated muscle fibers also produce signaling molecules that induce nearby motor neurons to sprout axon twigs to innervate the orphaned fiber (**Fig. 2**), which leads to enlarged motor units because then a single axon controls a greater number of motor fibers, as shown in **Fig. 1**B.

In myopathic disorders the pathology localizes to individual muscle fibers. Inflammatory or degenerative processes result in the loss of muscle fibers within the motor

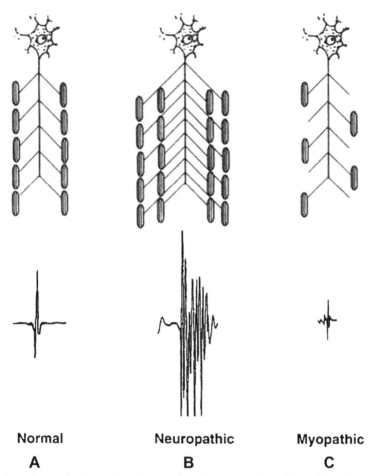

Normal   **Neuropathic**   **Myopathic**

A   **B**   **C**

Fig. 1. MUAP morphologies. (*A*) A normal motor unit. The unit consists of one motor neuron and all the muscle fibers it innervates. Below this is an example of how the MUAP might appear on the EMG screen. (*B*) Following reinnervation, the motor unit contains more muscle fibers, resulting in a MUAP that has longer duration and higher amplitude. (*C*) In a myopathic process muscle fibers within the motor units degenerate, leaving a smaller amplitude and shorter duration potential. (*Adapted from* Preston DC, Shapiro BE. Basic electromyography: analysis of motor unit action potentials. In: Electromyography and neuromuscular disorders: clinical-electrophysiologic correlations. 2nd edition. Philadelphia: Elsevier Butterworth Heinemann; 2005. p. 226; with permission.)

units, meaning that for any given motor unit there will be fewer muscle fibers activated with each propagated action potential. The motor units are smaller (see **Fig. 1**C).

Firing of a single motor neuron leads to the depolarization of many muscle fibers. If all of the muscle fibers in a motor unit depolarize at approximately the same time, their electric discharges will summate into a single potential seen on the EMG screen known as the motor unit action potential (MUAP), shown in **Fig. 1**A. The shape of the MUAP will change in characteristic ways in neuropathic and myopathic conditions, and these changes can be used to localize the pathology.

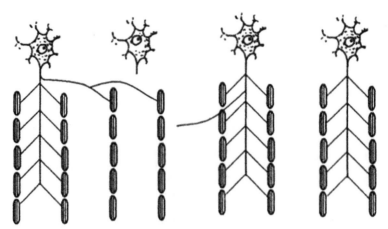

Fig. 2. Reinnervation. After a motor axon degenerates, it leaves the muscle fibers in its motor unit without innervation. The muscle fibers then produce trophic factors, which induce the neighboring neurons to reinnervate the orphaned fibers. (*Adapted from* Preston DC, Shapiro BE. Basic electromyography: analysis of motor unit action potentials. In: Electromyography and neuromuscular disorders: clinical-electrophysiologic correlations. 2nd edition. Philadelphia: Elsevier Butterworth Heinemann; 2005. p. 220; with permission.)

ELECTROMYOGRAPHY

Electromyography is the most important part of the electrodiagnostic evaluation of possible myopathy. A small needle is inserted into various muscles to measure voltage. The most commonly used type of needle electrode contains a small concentric, bipolar electrode that measures the electrical potential difference between the edge and the inside of the needle. The needle consists of a cannula with a strip of conducting material that is insulated except at the tip. The needle cannula serves as one electrode. The conducting material inside the cannula serves as the other electrode.[7] The concentric needle sizes range from 26 to 30 gauge and 2.5 to 5.0 cm in length. Within each muscle the needle must be moved several times to sample different locations within the muscle. With each movement the patient may feel a pinch similar to a blood draw. The electrical signal is amplified and then displayed on an oscilloscope screen in a plot of voltage versus time. The recording is converted to sound produced through a loudspeaker. Experienced electromyographers often rely on the audio characteristics when interpreting the results.

The number of muscles sampled varies based on the differential diagnosis. For example, testing for amyotrophic lateral sclerosis (ALS) will require sampling more muscles than carpal tunnel syndrome. Evaluation of a patient with myopathy depends on clinical history, but should include selected proximal muscles to establish a myopathic pattern as well as some more distal muscles to rule out a more diffuse process. In this case EMG might begin with proximal muscles such as deltoid, biceps, quadriceps, and iliopsoas as well any muscle identified as weak during the neurologic examination. The electromyographer samples each muscle in the relaxed state, in a state of voluntary contraction and maximal contraction. Thus, a patient must be able to follow simple instructions to obtain optimal results.

Voluntary Activity

The electrical activity of the motor units closest to the needle placement is evaluated. The morphology of the motor unit potentials gives information about whether a process is neuropathic or myopathic. Of course, the motor neurons must fire action potentials in order for motor units to appear on the screen. The simplest way to produce these potentials is to ask the patient to contract the muscle voluntarily. In chronic neuropathic conditions, the MUAPs are enlarged (see **Fig. 1**B), reflecting the expansion of the motor units themselves. After motor axons degenerate, neighboring motor neurons take over the orphaned muscle fibers. This takeover leads to higher amplitude motor units because the number of muscle fibers discharging simultaneously increases. The time duration of the MUAP also increases. The enlarged motor unit now covers a broader area of muscle tissue, so naturally more time is required to activate newly innervated fibers that are more distant than the native fibers. These characteristics come over the loudspeaker as a loud, dull thud. In myopathic processes the necrosis or apoptosis of muscle fibers leads to fewer muscle fibers in each motor unit, and produces motor units that appear small on EMG (see **Fig. 1**C). The duration of the MUAP is shorter than usual because some of the most distant muscle fibers have degenerated. These MUAPs sound like high-pitched crackling. In both types of conditions the action potential waveforms appear polyphasic. Polyphasia refers to the number of times the waveform crosses the baseline, which is an indication that muscle fibers are firing asynchronously. If all of the fibers fire together, the action potentials will summate and there will be few phases. Polyphasia can occur in both neuropathic and myopathic conditions.

Recruitment

The other important parameter to assess during voluntary contraction is recruitment. Initially, the single neuron fires repetitively at a slow rate as long as the force is maintained. If more force recruited, the single neuron will begin to fire more rapidly. This action is similar to rowing a boat—faster frequency of rowing produces more driving force. If still more force is recruited, additional motor neurons will begin to fire; this is known as recruitment. The force produced by a muscle is a function of the number of motor units firing and the frequency at which they fire. Force can be increased either by recruiting additional motor units or by increasing the frequency of the units already firing. Normally the ratio between number of motor units firing and firing rate is 1:5. Once a single unit begins firing at 10 Hz, another will begin to fire. At about 15 Hz there will be 3 units firing, and so on.[5] In this way additional motor units are recruited to increase the force generated. In neuropathic conditions there are fewer neurons and thus fewer motor units available, so recruitment is decreased. Thus, increased force is produced by driving the motor units to fire faster; this is known as decreased recruitment. In myopathic conditions there are normal numbers of motor units, but each individual unit is weaker than it would normally be. Thus, additional motor units are recruited at lower levels of force than they normally would be; this is known as early recruitment. The electromyographer will attempt to assess the recruitment pattern as normal, decreased, or early.

Spontaneous Activity

Electrical discharges that occur spontaneously in relaxed muscle can be useful for determining if there is pathologic condition and whether it localizes to muscle or peripheral nerve.

Normal spontaneous activity and insertional activity

During the evaluation the patient is asked to relax the muscle and the electromyographer evaluates spontaneous activity. Normal muscles produce spontaneous discharges for less than 2 seconds after each needle movement, due to the disruption of muscle fiber membranes by the needle; this is known as insertional activity. If it persists longer than 2 seconds, it is abnormally increased and is a nonspecific finding that may be caused by neuropathic or myopathic conditions. After insertional activity dissipates, normal muscle fibers are electrically silent except in certain regions located near the endplate of the neuromuscular junction. Here spontaneous electrical activity known as miniature endplate potentials (MEPP) and end-plate spikes (EPS) can be recorded in normal muscle.[8] MEPP are low-amplitude, short-duration discharges that correspond to the spontaneous release of a single vesicle of acetylcholine at the endplate. MEPP occur continuously and overlap one another, giving an audio quality like listening to a sound of the ocean in a seashell. EPS are higher amplitude spikes with waveform morphology similar to fibrillation. The difference is that EPS are irregular, whereas fibrillations fire rhythmically. The physiologic generator of EPS is controversial. One hypothesis is that EPS measure discharges from intramuscular nerves.[9] Alternatively, muscle spindles contain small muscle fibers that regulate the sensitivity of the proprioceptive apparatus. These intrafusal muscle fibers are innervated by a separate set of gamma motor neurons, not by the alpha motor neurons that innervate skeletal muscle. Some investigators have postulated that these intrafusal muscle fibers may be the origin of EPS.[10] In summary, therefore, there are 3 types of spontaneous activity seen in normal muscles: insertional activity, MEPP, and EPS.

Abnormal spontaneous activity

Other spontaneous discharges are abnormal. Their morphology can be useful in determining the source of the pathology. Abnormal spontaneous activity will originate from one of two sources: individual muscle fibers or peripheral nerve axons. The size and morphology of the electrical potential suggests the source of the abnormality. A discharge originating in a single muscle fiber will be small relative to a discharge of a single motor neuron. An abnormal discharge in the motor neuron will propagate down its axon to activate all the muscle fibers in the motor unit, possibly as many as hundreds of muscle fibers. Therefore, discharges originating from a peripheral nerve axon will be higher amplitude and longer duration than those originating from a single muscle fiber. As might be imagined, discharges originating from the peripheral nerve will be indistinguishable from the morphology of motor unit potentials that were voluntarily initiated. The muscle acts the same whether the action potential originates normally in the brain or pathologically due to hyperexcitable peripheral nerves. The difference is that motor units firing under voluntary control tend to fire slower and more irregularly than those originating from pathologic peripheral nerves.

Abnormalities originating in muscle fibers

Abnormal spontaneous discharges originating from the muscle fibers include fibrillation, positive sharp waves, complex repetitive discharges (CRDs), and myotonia.

Fibrillation A fibrillation is the spontaneous firing of a single muscle fiber,[11] and results when a muscle fiber is disconnected from the motor neuron. Fibrillation of skeletal muscle is not visible through the skin surface, and is detectable only by electrodiagnostic testing. The EMG appearance of fibrillation is a low-amplitude, short-duration potential with an initial negative deflection (**Fig. 3**). Fibrillation typically repeats in a rhythmic pattern, but can also occur irregularly.[12] The exact mechanism producing fibrillations is not known, but several hypotheses have been proposed.[13,14] In fibrillating muscle fibers there are local segments of abnormal muscle fiber membrane that are probably not more than millimeters in length. These abnormal regions are the origin of fibrillation potentials. Such abnormal segments most often occur near the neuromuscular junction, but can occur anywhere along the length of the muscle

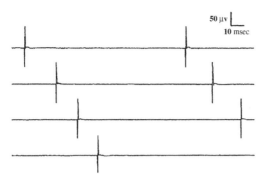

Fig. 3. Fibrillations. These are potentials of small amplitude and brief duration, and result from a single muscle fiber. The rhythmicity and morphology identifies them as fibrillation. Each potential appears the same, suggesting it is the same fiber discharging repetitively. (*Adapted from* Preston DC, Shapiro BE. Basic electromyography: analysis of spontaneous activity. In: Electromyography and neuromuscular disorders: clinical-electrophysiologic correlations. 2nd edition. Philadelphia: Elsevier Butterworth Heinemann; 2005. p. 205; with permission.)

fiber. Random, spontaneous depolarization of these abnormal segments that is sufficient to trigger an action potential results in irregular fibrillation. By contrast, rhythmic fibrillation is produced by regular, oscillating fluctuations in membrane potential. These spontaneous depolarizations and oscillating potentials may be caused by altered sodium conductance in the abnormal segment of membrane. Although denervated muscle fibers exhibit altered expression of acetylcholine receptors compared with a normal muscle fiber, fibrillations are probably not caused solely by hypersensitivity to circulating acetylcholine because fibrillation persists in the presence of tubocurare.

Fibrillation is typically evidence of a neuropathic disorder, although there are some exceptions. Certain myopathic processes, particularly inflammatory myopathies or certain muscular dystrophies, can develop fibrillation. Such fibrillation may be caused by inflammatory damage to the distal motor axon that makes the terminal branches of the nerve hyperexcitable. Alternatively, segmental necrosis may occur between the insertion or origin of the fiber and its neuromuscular junction, effectively severing the distal part of the fiber from its endplate.[15] Certain muscular dystrophies including Duchenne muscular dystrophy[16] and limb girdle muscular dystrophies also cause segmental necrosis and fibrillation. Furthermore, fibrillation can be seen in multifocal motor neuronopathy, which is a demyelinating condition in which the axon is typically preserved.

Positive sharp waves Positive sharp waves are a second type of spontaneous activity. Like fibrillation, positive sharp waves are also low-amplitude, short-duration, very regular discharges arising from a hyperexcitable muscle fiber. The clinical significance of positive sharp waves is usually the same as that of fibrillation—it suggests denervation.[15] Indeed, changing the needle position slightly often will convert a positive sharp wave into a fibrillation.

Complex repetitive discharges A third type of spontaneous activity arising from muscle is a CRD. CRDs are long volleys of potentials of uniform amplitude and frequency that start and stop abruptly.[17] On the loudspeaker these discharges sound like a mechanical hum, and may last minutes or up to half an hour in isolated cases.

CRDs originate with ephaptic transmission of action potentials from one diseased muscle fiber to the adjacent muscle fiber. The initiating muscle fiber discharges an action potential and then abnormally transmits the depolarization to its neighbor, which in turn transmits the depolarization to its neighbor. Eventually the process will come back to the original muscle fiber and begin again. This cycle creates the repetitive nature of the discharge. The process must originate and propagate in muscle fibers because CRDs are not abolished by curare or nerve block. CRDs are most often associated with chronic neuropathic disorders, although they can be seen in some myopathic diseases.[18] Loosely speaking and for practical purposes, then, CRDs may be thought of as a chronic form of fibrillation.

Myotonia The final type of spontaneous discharge originating in muscle fibers is myotonia. Myotonia is a repetitive firing of muscle fibers at high frequency. The morphology of myotonic discharges is a repetitive train of muscle fiber discharges. Occasionally the discharges may have a morphology similar to MUAP. Myotonic discharges are thought to result from unstable membranes in muscle fibers.[19] The frequency and amplitude of a myotonic discharge may fluctuate, giving it a waxing and waning sound over the loudspeaker that has been likened to a revving engine, motorcycle, or dive bomber. Myotonia must be differentiated from CRDs or neuromyotonia. CRDs have a steady sound, whereas myotonia waxes and wanes. Neuromyotonia does not have a waxing phase, but starts strong and dies out producing a "pinging" sound. The differential diagnosis of myotonia includes hereditary muscle diseases including myotonic dystrophy, paramyotonia congenita, myotonia congenita, hyperkalemic periodic paralysis, acid maltase deficiency, and other glycogen storage myopathies. It is also seen in some acquired muscle diseases such as hypothyroidism, colchicine toxicity, statin myopathy, and rarely in inflammatory myopathies.[20] Rarely, myotonia will also occur in any neuropathic condition that causes fibrillation.[21]

Abnormalities originating in peripheral nerve
There are 5 types of spontaneous activity arising from the peripheral nerve axon: fasciculation, grouped discharges, myokymia, cramp discharges, and neuromyotonia. Each of these discharges has the morphology of a MUAP on the EMG screen, because the abnormality originates in the motor axon. The difference between these types of discharges is the frequency at which they fire. The mechanism is thought to be destabilized, hypopolarized, or hyperexcitable motor neuron membranes.[22]

Fasciculation Fasciculation results from a single, spontaneous discharge that arises anywhere along the motor axon from the spinal cord to the terminal nerve twigs.[22,23] Clinically, fasciculations are spontaneous twitching of a small segment of muscle that is seen under the skin's surface. The morphology on the EMG screen is similar to that of a MUAP (**Fig. 4**), and it has an audio quality like a dull thud.

Although fibrillation and fasciculation both occur in motor neuron disease, they result from distinct pathophysiological processes. A fibrillation is not just a fasciculation that is too small to be seen from the skin's surface. The two types of discharges are generated from different sites in the neuraxis, that is, fibrillations in muscle fibers and fasciculations in neurons. Fibrillations are typically rhythmic, whereas fasciculation occurs irregularly. The former is caused by loss of innervation, but the latter presupposes intact innervation. The difference between fibrillation and fasciculation is important for the correct interpretation of EMG results.

Fasciculation is not always evidence of pathology. Repetitive clinical fasciculations can be seen in normal individuals, particularly during times of stress or fatigue. Isolated fasciculations are not uncommonly seen during EMG in normal individuals.

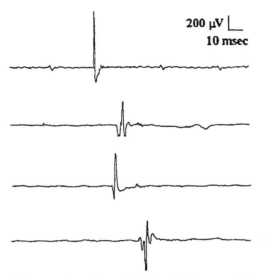

Fig. 4. Fasciculations. These are irregular potentials with the morphology of a motor unit. The vertical scale is 4 times that of **Fig. 3** showing fibrillations. Each potential appears different, indicating a different motor axon has fired. (*Adapted from* Preston DC, Shapiro BE. Basic electromyography: analysis of spontaneous activity. In: Electromyography and neuromuscular disorders: clinical-electrophysiologic correlations. 2nd edition. Philadelphia: Elsevier Butterworth Heinemann; 2005. p. 209; with permission.)

The duration and amplitude of these benign fasciculations appear similar to that of normal MUAPs. By contrast, fasciculations associated with ALS will have a neuropathic morphology on EMG (see **Fig. 1**B), and will occur in the context of other denervating features such as fibrillation or positive sharp waves.

Grouped discharge Four more types of spontaneous activity that can be thought of as variants of fasciculation are now discussed. A motor unit that fires 2, 3, or multiple times in a row is called a doublet, triplet, or multiplet. Together these are known as grouped discharges, which can be thought of as multiple fasciculations firing in a burst. The loudspeaker produces a sound like that of a machine gun firing a short burst. The clinical significance is the same as for fasciculations. In addition, grouped discharges are characteristically seen in hypocalcemia-induced tetany.[21]

Myokymia Myokymia is the term for bursts of discharges from a single motor unit that repeat regularly every 1 to 30 seconds. The loudspeaker emits a sound like marching soldiers. On EMG myokymia appears similar to grouped discharges, except the bursts repeat. Within a burst the discharges range from 5 to 150 times per second. Clinical myokymia refers to involuntary, undulating, or quivering muscle movements that look like snakes crawling under the skin. Myokymia classically is associated with radiation-induced plexitis or, less commonly, radiation-induced myeleopathy.[24] The differential diagnosis of myokymia also includes radiculopathy, gold intoxication, and channelopathies such as Isaac syndrome, periodic paralysis with myokymia, and rattlesnake envenomization. Myokymia has been reported in carpal tunnel syndrome.[24] Facial myokymia can occasionally be seen in disorders of the central nervous system that affect the facial nerve lower motor neurons as they exit the central nervous system, including pontine tumors or multiple sclerosis.

Cramp Cramps are spontaneous, painful, involuntary muscle contractions. On EMG a single motor unit is seen firing irregularly at high frequencies in the range of 40 to 150 Hz. A cramp may be thought of loosely as continuous myokymia. The morphology on EMG resembles a motor unit rather than a muscle fiber, because perhaps surprisingly cramps originate from peripheral nerves rather than the muscle itself.

Neuromyotonia Neuromyotonia results from prolonged high-frequency (150–300 Hz) discharges from a single motor axon. The amplitude and frequency decrease throughout the discharge, leading to a characteristic pinging sound. Unlike myotonia, neuromyotonia originates from the motor axon and does not have an upstroke or revving sound. It is classically associated with acquired neuromyotonia, which is also known as Isaac syndrome. It is important to distinguish neuromyotonia from myotonia because the differential diagnosis of each is vastly different.

The spectrum of peripheral nerve hyperexcitability The 5 types of abnormal spontaneous activity originating in the motor axon that are discussed here form a spectrum of peripheral nerve hyperexcitability. The physiologic source generator for each is the same, but moving up the spectrum from fasciculation to neuromyotonia the discharges of the motor neuron become more continuous and occur at higher frequency. The primary difference between cramps, for example, and fasciculations is that the former betrays a more excitable nerve than the latter.

Fasciculation may be seen in some muscle diseases if the distal axons twigs are involved. In general, however, EMG evidence of peripheral nerve hyperexcitability argues against the diagnosis of primary muscle disease. As always, the entire clinical picture must be considered.

Single-Fiber EMG

Single-fiber EMG is a technique that attempts to isolate 2 muscle fibers in the same motor unit to determine whether there is an abnormality at the neuromuscular junction. In a patient with suspected myopathy single-fiber EMG is not usually indicated, so a complete discussion of single-fiber EMG is beyond the scope of this article. Although it can be helpful in ruling out diseases of the neuromuscular junction as a cause of weakness, standard EMG, repetitive nerve conduction studies, clinical history, and antibody testing are usually adequate to differentiate these disorders from myopathy.

Complications

EMG is an invasive procedure, and although complications are rare it is important for patients to be aware of them. Local muscle ache in the examined muscles is the most common adverse effect of the procedure. Ache can be treated with over-the-counter analgesics. More serious complications, such as infection or bleeding, occur rarely. Sterile procedures are similar to those required for drawing blood—the skin is sufficiently cleaned with an alcohol swab. Bleeding complications can be minimized by employing a small needle, and most muscles tested in a standard EMG are easily compressible. Thus, treatment with warfarin or hemophilia is not a contraindication to EMG, but severe thrombocytopenia may be a relative contraindication. Transmission of blood-borne pathogens is easily prevented by using a new disposable needle with every patient. There are more serious risks with certain muscles such as the diaphragm, rhomboids, or abdominal muscles, which require care to avoid pneumothorax or infectious peritonitis. These muscles are not routinely tested, however. One practical consequence of disrupting the muscle with the needle is that the serum creatine kinase (CK) will increase. In one study the CK was elevated in up to 30% of healthy volunteers between 4 and 48 hours following EMG.[25] The mean CK at its peak was 178% of baseline and did not exceed 161 IU/L.

Technical Factors

The interpretation of EMG involves a degree of subjectivity. There are a variety of technical factors that can influence the results. The duration of MUAPs, the degree of polyphasia, and the presence of fibrillations may vary based on the temperature[15,26,27] and age[27,28] of the patient as well as the particular muscle.[5,29] The morphology of the MUAP waveform also depends on distance of the motor unit from the recording electrode. An inexperienced examiner may mistake distant units for neuropathic ones. Excessive noise from nearby electrical equipment can obscure faint fibrillation, or 60-cycle interference can sound like a complex repetitive discharge. Not surprisingly, the quality of the study is determined by the level of experience of the electromyographer. Patients sometimes have difficulty tolerating the entire examination, but a seasoned practitioner will be able to keep the patient at ease long enough to collect all of the necessary data. The electromyographer must select the appropriate muscles to sample on-the-fly based on the results of nerve conduction studies (NCS) and needle EMG of muscles already done. This approach requires detailed knowledge of peripheral neuroanatomy. Moreover, the electromyographer must be sure the needle has been inserted into the correct muscle. For example, the flexor digitorum profundus is divided into median and ulnar heads, but these muscles lie on top of one another. It would be easy to stick the needle too deeply and record from the ulnar innervated muscle when the median innervated muscle was intended. Care must be taken to avoid sampling error, because the disease pathology may be patchy. Finding normal motor units in one area of muscle does not guarantee that the entire muscle is normal. There is also room for error in interpreting the type of discharges that appear on the screen. Neuromyotonia and myotonia are similar, but the diagnostic implications of each are quite different. Normal miniature endplate potentials could be confused with abnormal fibrillation. CRDs can be confused with myotonia.

Summary

EMG can often differentiate neuropathic from myopathic conditions (**Table 1**). Neuropathic conditions typically show long-duration, high-amplitude MUAPs and decreased recruitment during voluntary contraction and fibrillation during the relaxed state. Myopathic conditions typically show short-duration, low-amplitude MUAPs with early recruitment, and may or may not have fibrillation. These principles govern the majority of cases, but there are some exceptions. For example, during the early phases of reinnervation after a severe peripheral nerve transection, nascent regenerating motor units may appear small on EMG, mimicking a myopathic condition.[20] On the other hand, long-duration polyphasic MUAPs have been reported in chronic polymyositis and Becker muscular dystrophy.[30] This finding underscores the limitation of electrophysiologic studies in making a definitive diagnosis of muscle disease.

NERVE CONDUCTION STUDIES

NCS typically are also performed when a physician refers a patient to an electrophysiologist for "EMG." NCS are usually performed to evaluate both motor and sensory nerves. A recording electrode is placed over either the peripheral nerve itself or a muscle stimulated by the peripheral nerve to be tested. The electrical potential at this electrode is compared with a reference electrode placed over electrical neutral

Table 1
Characteristics of EMG findings in myopathic and neuropathic conditions

	Myopathic	Neuropathic
Voluntary Activity		
Motor unit action potential		
Duration	Decreased	Increased
Amplitude	Decreased	Increased
Polyphasia	Increased	Increased
Recruitment	Early	Decreased
Spontaneous Activity		
Fibrillations/Positive sharp waves	Present in some conditions	Present
Myotonia	Present in some conditions	Rare
Complex repetitive discharges	Rare	Occasionally (if chronic)
Peripheral nerve hyperexcitability	Rare	Occasionally

tissue such as bone or tendon. An electrical device then stimulates the peripheral nerve at a more proximal location. The stimulation depolarizes the axon and initiates an action potential, which then conducts down the nerve axon toward the electrodes. As the electrical charge passes under the recording electrode, the potential difference is measured on the oscilloscope.

NCS primarily evaluate the function of peripheral nerves, and thus are not particularly relevant in producing positive evidence for primary muscle disease. One might think, however, that motor NCS would provide some information. In motor NCS, the recording electrode is placed over a muscle innervated by the nerve to be studied (eg, abductor pollicis brevis in a median motor study). The electrical discharges detected by the oscilloscope in this case are discharges of muscle fibers, not nerve axons. The nerve is stimulated, creating a depolarization of the axon at the site of stimulation. The resultant action potential travels down the axon, then down all of the axon twigs, triggering release of acetylcholine at all of the neuromuscular junctions within the motor unit. Then all of the muscle fibers in the motor unit depolarize, and this potential is detected by the machine; this is called a compound motor action potential (CMAP). This setup is different to that of sensory NCS. Because sensory nerves do not fire muscle fibers, the electrical activity must be recorded over the nerve axons themselves. Why are motor nerves tested differently to sensory nerves? In normal individuals each motor axon produces many electrical discharges from muscle fibers, and thus the signal will be amplified naturally. This process increases the signal-to-noise ratio.

Motor NCS are often normal in myopathies. This seems counterintuitive, because motor NCS record electrical activity in muscles, which is the site of pathology in primary muscle disease. One might expect that the CMAP amplitude would be lower, because there are fewer viable muscle fibers available to discharge. However, usually distal hand and foot muscles are tested, and these are often affected by muscle diseases only late in the course. If proximal muscles are tested or in specific conditions affecting distal muscles such as inclusion body myositis, CMAP amplitude may be decreased.[1] But a decreased CMAP amplitude is more commonly caused by conditions other than primary muscle disease. For these reasons other tests, including needle EMG, are more useful in diagnosing primary muscle disease, especially at early stages.

Although NCS do not typically provide positive evidence for primary muscle disease, they are useful in ruling out other causes of weakness including brachial or lumbosacral plexopathy, demyelinating or axonal neuropathy, and diseases of the neuromuscular junction. Myasthenia gravis, acute and chronic inflammatory demyelinating polyradiculoneuropathy, and diabetic amyotrophy are common causes of weakness and may be diagnosed with NCS.

REPETITIVE STIMULATION

Repetitive stimulation is performed to evaluate the neuromuscular junction. It is not routinely performed in the evaluation of myopathy except to rule out conditions such as myasthenia gravis (MG) and Lambert-Eaton myasthenic syndrome (LEMS) as a cause of weakness. The diagnostic setup is the same as that for routine NCS. The difference is that electrical stimulation is administered to the nerve repetitively at low frequencies of 2 to 3 times per second. In disorders of the neuromuscular junction, the CMAP will decrease with repetitive stimulation at low frequencies. Usually a distal nerve is tested to minimize discomfort (eg, ulnar). If this is normal, more proximal muscles including the trapezius or facial nerve are tested. If a decrement of CMAP amplitude at low frequency occurs, nerve conductions are repeated after exercise (several minutes of vigorous contraction of the tested muscle) to differentiate MG from LEMS.

CASE PRESENTATION

Ms. A is a 43-year-old woman who presents with muscle weakness. About 4 months ago she began to experience myalgias and muscle tenderness in her thighs. Two months later she noticed difficulty holding her arms over her head when she fixes her hair and difficulty climbing a flight of stairs without using the railing. Just recently she began to have difficulty swallowing lettuce. She has occasional muscle cramps but no muscle twitching. She denies paresthesias or numbness. She does not have a rash. She does not smoke cigarettes and drinks alcohol on social occasions. Family history is significant for her paternal grandmother who died suddenly in her sleep at age 53 years. She had been using a walker at that time.

On examination, she had no rash or lesions on her fingertips. Speech was normal. Cranial nerves were significant for mild weakness of the facial muscles and sternocleidomastoid. There was no ptosis. She had weakness of the neck flexors, neck extensors, deltoid, biceps, triceps, hip flexors, and knee flexors. She was unable to arise from a chair without using her arms, and had difficulty walking on her toes. Reflexes were hypoactive. Plantar responses were flexor bilaterally. She had a waddling gait.

Laboratory testing was significant for CK of 2154. Electrolytes and complete blood count were normal. A liver profile revealed an elevated aspartate aminotransferase and alanine aminotransferase. EMG showed increased insertional activity, moderate fibrillation, small polyphasic MUAPs, and early recruitment.

Discussion

EMG findings point to a myopathic process. Small polyphasic MUAPs occur because individual muscle fibers degenerate randomly, leaving motor units smaller. This situation contrasts with neuropathic conditions such as ALS, chronic inflammatory demyelinating polyradiculoneuropathy, or polyradiculopathy, in which motor units become larger as the remaining neurons take over orphaned muscle fibers. Early recruitment indicates that individual motor units are weak, so more motor units than would normally be required must be recruited to produce adequate force. Fibrillation is a typically a sign of denervation, but can be seen in some primary muscle diseases including polymyositis, inclusion body myositis, or muscular dystrophy. The elevated CK similarly confirm a primary muscle disease. Although CK may be mildly elevated in some neuropathic conditions including ALS, it would not typically reach the level seen in this case.

The differential diagnosis at this point includes inflammatory myopathies (polymyositis or dermatomyositis) and muscular dystrophies (limb girdle muscular dystrophy). The pattern of weakness is not typical for inclusion body myositis, which often begins with knee extensors and finger flexors. Polymyalgia rheumatica does not cause abnormal CK or EMG. Inherited muscular dystrophies are certainly a consideration given the patient's family history. Her grandmother was using a walker at an early age and may have died of a cardiac arrhythmia, which is associated with many muscular dystrophies. Becker muscular dystrophy is an adult-onset muscular dystrophy that is X-linked, and so does not usually affect females. Myotonic dystrophy type 1 is the most common adult-onset muscular dystrophy, but tends to affect distal muscles. Myotonic dystrophy type 2 affects proximal muscles preferentially, but would be associated with myotonia on EMG. Limb girdle muscular dystrophy is a heterogeneous group of inherited muscular dystrophies that cause proximal muscle weakness, which can be inherited in an autosomal dominant or autosomal recessive pattern. A muscle biopsy is indicated to make a specific diagnosis, which shows endomysial inflammation with invasion of non-necrotic fibers, and internal nuclei, myofiber necrosis, atrophy, and regeneration. Immunohistochemical staining for proteins associated with several limb girdle muscular dystrophies was negative. These findings are consistent with a diagnosis of polymyositis.

SUMMARY

Electrodiagnostic testing can be useful in differentiating primary muscle disorders from other causes of weakness. NCS are important for ruling out causes of weakness localizing to nerve roots, plexus, peripheral nerves, or neuromuscular junction. EMG detects primary muscle disorders but also differentiates myopathic from neuropathic diseases. Neuropathic and myopathic processes each produce characteristic changes in the pattern of electrical discharges in muscle tissue. In many cases electrodiagnostic testing does not produce a specific diagnosis, but can determine who would be a candidate for further invasive or expensive testing. Because of many technical factors and matters of subjective interpretation, it is important that an experienced electromyographer perform the testing.

REFERENCES

1. Wilbourn AJ. The electrodiagnostic examination with myopathies. J Clin Neurophysiol 1993;10(2):132–48.
2. Danon MJ, Schliselfeld LH. Study of skeletal muscle glycogenolysis and glycolysis in chronic steroid myopathy, non-steroid histochemical type-2 fiber atrophy, and denervation. Clin Biochem 2007;40(1/2):46–51.
3. Afifi AK, Bergman RA, Harvey JC. Steroid myopathy. Clinical, histologic and cytologic observations. Johns Hopkins Med J 1968;123(4):158–73.
4. Dekhuijzen PN, Decramer M. Steroid-induced myopathy and its significance to respiratory disease: a known disease rediscovered. Eur Respir J 1992;5(8): 997–1003.
5. Preston DC, Shapiro BE. Basic electromyography: analysis of motor unit action potentials. In: Electromyography and neuromuscular disorders: clinical-electrophysiologic

correlations. 2nd edition. Philadelphia: Elsevier Butterworth Heinemann; 2005. p. 215–29.

6. Engel WK. Focal myopathic changes produced by electromyographic and hypodermic needles. "Needle myopathy". Arch Neurol 1967;16(5):509–11.

7. Gitter AJ, Stolov WC. AAEM minimonograph #16: instrumentation and measurement in electrodiagnostic medicine–Part I. Muscle Nerve 1995;18(8):799–811.

8. Buchthal F, Rosenfalck P. Spontaneous electrical activity of human muscle. Electroencephalogr Clin Neurophysiol 1966;20(4):321–36.

9. Jones RV Jr, Lambert EH, Sayre GP. Source of a type of insertion activity in electromyography with evaluation of a histologic method of localization. Arch Phys Med Rehabil 1955;36(5):301–10.

10. Partanen J. End plate spikes in the human electromyogram. Revision of the fusimotor theory. J Physiol Paris 1999;93(1/2):155–66.

11. Li CL, Shy GM, Wells J. Some properties of mammalian skeletal muscle fibres with particular reference to fibrillation potentials. J Physiol 1957;135(3):522–35.

12. Smith JW, Thesleff S. Spontaneous activity in denervated mouse diaphragm muscle. J Physiol 1976;257(1):171–86.

13. Purves D, Sakmann B. Membrane properties underlying spontaneous activity of denervated muscle fibres. J Physiol 1974;239(1):125–53.

14. Thesleff S, Ward MR. Studies on the mechanism of fibrillation potentials in denervated muscle. J Physiol 1975;244(2):313–23.

15. Desmedt JE. Muscular dystrophy contrasted with denervation: different mechanisms underlying spontaneous fibrillations. Electroencephalogr Clin Neurophysiol Suppl 1978;34:531–46.

16. Desmedt JE, Borenstein S. Regeneration in Duchenne muscular dystrophy. Electromyographic evidence. Arch Neurol 1976;33(9):642–50.

17. Emeryk B, Hausmanowa-Petrusewicz I, Nowak T. Spontaneous volleys of bizarre high-frequency potentials (b.h.f.p.) in neuro-muscular diseases. Part II. An analysis of the morphology of spontaneous volleys of bizarre high-frequency potentials in neuro-muscular diseases. Electromyogr Clin Neurophysiol 1974;14(4):339–54.

18. Stoehr M. Low frequency bizarre discharges. A particular type of electromyographical spontaneous activity in paretic skeletal muscle. Electromyogr Clin Neurophysiol 1978;18(2):147–56.

19. Ptacek LJ, Johnson KJ, Griggs RC. Genetics and physiology of the myotonic muscle disorders. N Engl J Med 1993;328(7):482–9.

20. Amato AA, Russell JA. Testing in neuromuscular disease—electrodiagnosis and other modalities. In: Neuromuscular disorders. New York: McGraw-Hill; 2008. p. 17–69.

21. Preston DC, Shapiro BE. Basic electromyography: analysis of spontaneous activity. In: Electromyography and neuromuscular disorders: clinical-electrophysiologic correlations. 2nd edition. Philadelphia: Elsevier Butterworth Heinemann; 2005. p. 199–213.

22. Roth G. The origin of fasciculations. Ann Neurol 1982;12(6):542–7.

23. Wettstein A. The origin of fasciculations in motoneuron disease. Ann Neurol 1979; 5(3):295–300.

24. Albers JW, Allen AA 2nd, Bastron JA, et al. Limb myokymia. Muscle Nerve 1981; 4(6):494–504.

25. Levin R, Pascuzzi RM, Bruns DE, et al. The time course of creatine kinase elevation following concentric needle EMG. Muscle Nerve 1987;10(3):242–5.

26. Denys EH. AAEM minimonograph #14: the influence of temperature in clinical neurophysiology. Muscle Nerve 1991;14(9):795–811.

27. Buchthal F, Pinell P, Rosenfalck P. Action potential parameters in normal human muscle and their physiological determinants. Acta Physiol Scand 1954;32(2/3): 219–29.
28. Sacco G, Buchthal F, Rosenfalck P. Motor unit potentials at different ages. Arch Neurol 1962;6:366–73.
29. Kraft GH. Decay of fibrillation potential amplitude following nerve injury. Electro-encephalogr Clin Neurophysiol 1985;60:105P.
30. Uncini A, Lange DJ, Lovelace RE, et al. Long-duration polyphasic motor unit potentials in myopathies: a quantitative study with pathological correlation. Muscle Nerve 1990;13(3):263–7.

Molecular Diagnosis of Myopathies

Andrew Gomez-Vargas, MD, PhD, Steven K. Baker, MSc, MD, FRCP(C)*

KEYWORDS

- Restriction fragment length polymorphism
- Polymerase chain reaction
- Allele specific oligonucleotide analysis

Rapid and accurate diagnosis of diseases is very important for the appropriate treatment of patients. Recent advances at the molecular level and detection technologies are upgrading clinical diagnostics by providing new ways of diagnosis, with higher speed and accuracy. The recently developed molecular diagnostic assays based on the amplification, restriction maps, or hybridization of probe nucleic acids with target nucleic acids from clinical samples are allowing effective detection of various diseases with higher sensitivity and specificity compared with the other techniques used to date. Several applications of DNA microarrays for diagnosing specific diseases have been reported: genotyping and determination of disease-relevant genes or disease-causative agents, mutation analysis using relatively low-density DNA microarrays, single nucleotide polymorphisms (SNPs) screening using high-density DNA microarrays, analysis of copy number changes at the level of chromosome using comparative genomic hybridization DNA microarrays (arrayCGH), and global determination of posttranslational modifications including methylation, acetylation, and alternative splicing. Molecular genetic advances are creating a dynamic state of ever-expanding disease classifications for inherited and metabolic neuromuscular disease. Early neuromuscular disease classification systems were predicated on clinical features and patterns of inheritance. However, the nomenclature used to categorize various disease phenotypes is inconsistent, because some may be subclassified according to age of disease onset whereas others may be subclassified according to electrodiagnostic features.

Neuromuscular diseases (NMD) constitute a group of phenotypically and genetically heterogeneous disorders, characterized by (progressive) weakness and atrophy of proximal and/or distal muscles. The objective of molecular testing is to confirm the pathogenicity of a relevant sequence variation by correlating an individual's phenotype with what is expected in a given condition. If a novel nonsynonymous mutation

The authors have nothing to disclose.
Department of Medicine, McMaster University, 1200 Main Street West, HSC 2H22, Hamilton, ON, Canada L8 N 3Z5
* Corresponding author.
E-mail address: bakersk@mcmaster.ca

Rheum Dis Clin N Am 37 (2011) 269–287
doi:10.1016/j.rdc.2011.01.009
0889-857X/11/$ – see front matter © 2011 Elsevier Inc. All rights reserved.

rheumatic.theclinics.com

is identified then possible pathogenicity is determined by genotype-phenotype correlations within the family, if this is possible. Software programs such as Polyphen and SIFT offer first-pass assessments of whether the mutation would be tolerated by the protein, but these are only proxy estimates of pathogenicity.[1] However, clinical diagnosis based on physical examination, family history, and noninvasive procedures is very important for the comprehensive evaluation of patients with NMDs, and molecular testing does not replace it.

Molecular diagnosis of NMDs is based on the nature of the sequence variation and the specifics of the genomic changes under consideration that dictate the method used for the investigation. For example, large variations, such as duplication of a segment of a chromosome as present in Charcot-Marie-Tooth disease type IA, are visible with appropriate labeling methods under a microscope, whereas small variations, such as a single base pair substitutions or mutations, might require sequencing for detection. For autosomal-recessive and X-linked disorders, diagnostic testing methods can be different for symptomatic individuals than for carriers, if the method only determines the presence, not the quantity, of mutant alleles (**Table 1**).

Table 1
Common techniques in molecular diagnosis

Method	Description	Advantages/Disadvantages
Chromosome		
Fluorescent in situ hybridization (FISH)	Visualization of normal/ abnormal DNA sequences	Detects mosaicism
DNA[a]		
Restriction fragments (RFLP)	DNA fragments separated by electrophoresis	Requires mutation in restriction site to be known
PCR used with other techniques	Creates multiple DNA copies	Does not detect different mutations from each other
Sequencing	Gets DNA detail sequence	Does not detect deletions/ duplications
Denaturing techniques (DGGE, SSCP)	Short DNA segments separated by mobility	Does not distinguish between polymorphism and mutation
Protein truncation test	In vitro gene expression	Detects non-sense mutations
mRNA		
Northern blot	Separates mRNA	Determines cell type DNA expression
Microarray expression analysis	Quantifies mRNA copies	Determines level of gene expression
Protein		
Immunohistochemistry	Antibodies against target protein	All of them might be biased because enzymatic defect
Enzyme functional analysis	Protein activity	can be the consequence of other protein defect
Western blot	Separates proteins by mobility	

Abbreviations: DGGE, denaturing gradient gel electrophoresis; PCR, polymerase chain reaction; RFLP, restriction fragment length polymorphism; SSCP, single-strand conformation polymorphism.
[a] DNA usually is genomic but mtDNA can be used. These test were explained in the first section of this article.

MODES OF INHERITANCE

Three different modalities of genetic transmission have been described for nuclear DNA. Autosomal recessive, in which the two different forms of the same gene (ie, alleles), each inherited from a different parent, are affected by a pathogenic mutation to cause the disease. For instance, an autosomal-recessive limb girdle muscular dystrophy (LGMD) in members with the same mutation present in the homozygous state (two copies). Autosomal dominant is the result of a mutation in a single gene or allele. Passing on the mutant allele transmits the disease to the offspring. A good example is autosomal-dominant tibial muscular dystrophy in members with heterozygous mutations (one copy), affecting the same gene that produces LGMD.[2] X-linked disorders are associated with mutation in the X-chromosome and might be compromising 1 or 2 alleles depending of the severity of the mutation. For example, some X-linked dystrophin and probably most GJB1 mutations (causing X-linked Charcot-Marie-Tooth disease) are symptomatic in females. These are very simple rules; however, to complicate genetic disorders it is becoming more clear that a single mutation can be associated with different phenotypes depending on other regulatory phenomena such as epigenetics; that is, hypomethylation may account for some patients with facioscapulohumeral muscular dystrophy (FSHD) who have no abnormalities in their genomic sequences[3] and environmental factors. Similarly, interaction between different mutated genes can have substantial consequences, in contrast to when only one of them is affected. For example, some mutations in the 3 collagen VI subunit genes (COL6A1, COL6A2, and COL6A3) produce autosomal-dominant Bethlem myopathy whereas other mutations in different locations in these genes produce autosomal-recessive Ullrich congenital muscular dystrophy.[4]

Mitochondrial inheritance is the asexual transmission of mtDNA from a mother to her children.[5] As all children of a woman inherit the same mtDNA sequence, there is generally in maternal inheritance a high recurrence risk in the future siblings of an affected child, often approaching 100%, although a high degree of clinical variability is common. Cells contain hundreds or thousands of mitochondria (skeletal muscle studies found a mean of 3650 mitochondrial genomes per 2 nuclear genomes) and each mitochondrion has multiple (estimates of 2–10) mtDNA genomes.[6] mtDNA point mutations that are present in blood do not always reach the threshold for clinical disease in some or all of the matrilineal relatives, who can be asymptomatic or oligosymptomatic.[7] Also, there are cases of nuclear DNA mutations affecting the protein activity of enzymes that play an important role in mitochondrial function. Around 100 nuclear genes have been described with mitochondrial functions, such as governing mitochondrial structure, function, replication, and protein import.[8] Therefore, mitochondrial disorders can also be autosomal dominant or recessive, for example, autosomal dominant progressive external ophthalmoplegia or autosomal recessive progressive external ophthalmoplegia.

LABORATORY INVESTIGATIONS

The diagnosis of inherited and metabolic disorders is challenging enough, and it is very difficult to confirm them based on clinical findings or routine chemistry analyses. Usually the evaluation of individuals at risk includes investigations such as biochemical, electrodiagnostic, histopathologic, and molecular studies. The purpose of this review is to focus on molecular diagnosis.

Molecular testing is useful in specific disorders in individuals with preliminary testing, suggesting the possibility of well-characterized disorders including conditions associated with point mutations, such as mitochondrial disorders like NARP (neuropathy, ataxia, and retinitis pigmentosa), MERRF (myoclonic epilepsy with ragged-red fibers), or MELAS (mitochondrial encephalopathy with lactic acidosis and stroke).[9]

DNA AND RNA INVESTIGATIONS

Molecular testing at this level for inherited disorders can be divided in 4 categories: prenatal, carrier, susceptibility testing, and diagnostic. Usually ordered to confirm a diagnosis and requiring in general just a blood sample, molecular investigations do not always reach an accuracy of 100%. In fact, disorders with single mutations that are not well characterized or associated with a particular disorder only explain 60% to 70% of the causative mutations; therefore, a negative result for these disorders does not completely rule out the diagnosis.

There are different methods used to detect known and novel mutations. To determine which particular method is better, it is important to determine the potential size of the defect, whether DNA or mRNA should be used, and the type of tissue to analyze. The physical principles explaining the differences between mutant and wild-type DNA are based on (1) differences in electrophoretic mobility, (2) the ability of restriction enzymes from bacteria to recognize specific sequences and cleavage the double-stranded DNA, and (3) inhibition of formation of DNA duplex hybrids with synthetic probes.

DETECTION OF KNOWN MUTANTS
Polymerase Chain Reaction

The 1993 Nobel Prize in Chemistry was awarded to Dr Kary B. Mullis for the invention of the polymerase chain reaction (PCR), a method that made it possible to copy a large number of DNA fragments in only a few hours. PCR can amplify very specific segments of the genome from 1 or 2 copies to a workable quantity of 1 million or more copies. An important limitation of PCR is that the size of a DNA segment that can be amplified, which is limited to approximately 3000 base pairs, typically significantly fewer. A classic example is the amplification of genes associated with FSHD and spinal muscular atrophy (SMA), 2 genes that are similar but differ in the surrounding sequences, therefore making it impossible to amplify a big enough fragment to differentiate between them. Similarly, it does not distinguish among the presence of 1, 2, or 3 copies, typically related with duplication of genes (**Fig. 1**).[10]

Restriction Fragment Length Polymorphism

Restriction fragment length polymorphism (RFLP) is a procedure based on the recognition of amplified genomic DNA of the allelic variation of DNA or mutant genotype by bacterial enzymes that recognize specific sequences of DNA, cutting them, and producing DNA fragments with different sizes, which can be further separated by electrophoresis. The recognition is based on uncleaved DNA fragment that was not recognized by the bacterial enzyme, giving the change in sequence.[11] Therefore, the mutant DNA will (ie, mutation causes new restriction site) or will not (ie, mutation causes loss of a restriction site) be cut by the restriction endonuclease. This differential pattern of cutting or generation of fragments of different lengths, when compared with the wild-type or normal DNA fragments, explains how this technique was named (**Fig. 2**).

Molecular Cytogenetics

These studies provided early "physical maps" of chromosomes, and allowed for the direct visual identification of many genetic diseases in which sequence variations

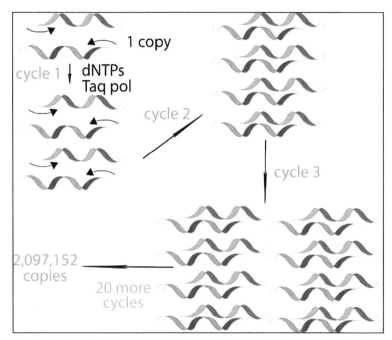

Fig. 1. Amplification of a DNA sequence by polymerase chain reaction (PCR). A target sequence is copied by the use of a forward and reverse primer, and repeated cycles of denaturing of double-stranded DNA, attachment of the primers, and copying by a polymerase, obtaining millions of copies of the same gene from the patient sample, thus allowing further characterization.

were of sufficient size to be recognized by abnormalities in the number, size, or pattern of bands present. Examples include various diseases with extra chromosomes (trisomies) or missing chromosomes. Molecular methods using chromosomal probes, complementary nucleic acid sequences binding directly to a short segment of

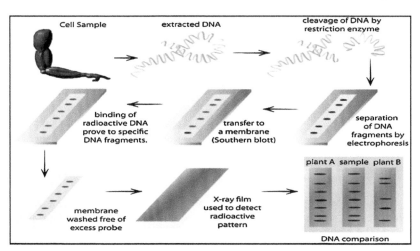

Fig. 2. Southern blot. dsDNA is fragmented by restriction enzymes, separated by gel electrophoresis, denatured to single-stranded DNA, and then probed.

a chromosome in defined location, produce higher resolution visualization. This technique, known as fluorescent in situ hybridization (FISH), uses fluorescent probes to detect sequence variations or mutants. This method has been applied to the diagnosis of CMT1A and hereditary neuropathy with liability to pressure palsy, disorders in which there is either a large duplication or deletion of a chromosomal segment, and for dystrophin analysis (**Fig. 3**).[12]

Allele-Specific Oligonucleotide Analysis

Allele-specific oligonucleotide analysis is based on amplification of DNA from the patient and hybridization with probes (oligonucleotides), each one of them testing for specific point mutations. It can evaluate up to 20 different point mutations in a target DNA. These probes, which are single-strand DNA, are immobilized in a solid support and then incubated with denatured DNA from the patient, in an attempt to find a complementary sequence that binds covalently to the probe. This methodology has proven to be more cost-effective than RFLP analysis, especially in analyzing mtDNA, because it can detect 18 different mtDNA point mutations simultaneously (**Fig. 4**).[13]

Sequencing

The goal is to determine the sequence of a specific gene base by base. This procedure is based on PCR amplification of patient's DNA, and the sample is run on a polyacrylamide electrophoresis gel able to separate fragments by size, even with just one base of difference, and determine the sequence of the gene.[14] Sometimes sequencing may result in diagnostic uncertainties when the gene of interest has highly similar sequences elsewhere in the genome (**Fig. 5**).[15]

New mutation detection

Denaturing gradient gel electrophoresis and temperature gradient gel electrophoresis These two similar techniques are based on the denaturing properties of DNA molecules. The extent of denaturation is dependent on its sequence, and it

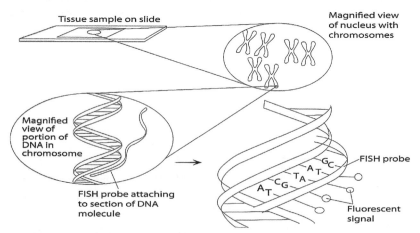

Fig. 3. Fluorescent in situ hybridization (FISH). Cells are partially denatured, combined with a fluorescent small nucleotide probe that is complementary to a target sequence, and then renatured. The chromosomes are then examined with fluorescent microscopy and the number of chromosomes with a target detected. This method is particularly useful for chromosomal deletions, duplications, or analysis of mosaicism, in which the numbers of alleles of a particular gene sequence within individual cells can be detected.

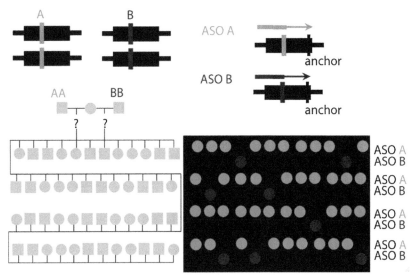

Fig. 4. Allele-specific oligonucleotide analysis. Allele-specific primers are designed (A, B) for each specific mutation affecting a particular gene. These probes are labeled with a detectable substance (ie, biotin) and hybridized to the wild type and mutant DNA on nylon membranes, and visualized by color development. As shown, it can be used to screen large number of samples.

varies with temperature and chemical conditions.[16] The amount of separation from double-stranded DNA to single-stranded DNA is inversely proportional to its mobility in gel electrophoresis. Whereas Denaturing gradient gel electrophoresis (DGGE) uses electrophoresis through a gradient of increasing chemical denaturant to separate different mutants of genes,[17] temperature gradient gel electrophoresis (TGGE) uses a temperature gradient analogously.[18] DGGE has been used for analysis of dystrophin mutations (**Fig. 6**).[19]

INDICATIONS FOR GENETIC TESTING IN NEUROMUSCULAR DISEASE

Specific indications for genetic testing are not clear. The following comprises a guide to decision-making specific to patients with neuromuscular disease. Genetic testing is always helpful in establishing the diagnosis, and if the result is negative it is helpful to redirect which kind of investigations should be ordered in the future. Genetic testing may be helpful in the management of patients. Although there is no cure for any inherited neuromuscular disease, there are treatments in the fullest meaning of this term. For example, ensuring close cardiac follow-up and monitoring for heart block with timely insertion of pacemakers in patients with myotonic dystrophy can be life saving, and prevents further unnecessary testing such as muscle biopsy or imaging studies. More importantly, it avoids non-necessary treatments previously seen, such as esophageal procedures in patients with myotonic dystrophy and oculopharyngeal muscular dystrophy, and lumbar laminectomies and orthopedic leg procedures in patients with inherited neuropathies (**Fig. 7**).

Applications

The current nomenclature system for inherited and metabolic myopathies is increasingly blurred by progress in their clinical and molecular understanding. For

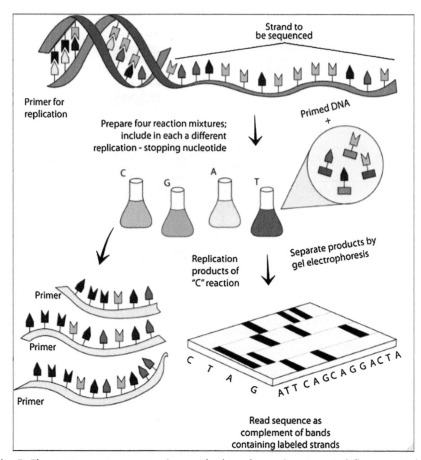

Fig. 5. The most common sequencing method used now is automated fluorescent dye-terminator sequencing. PCR with one forward primer is performed on genomic or cDNA, incorporating a mixture of dideoxynucleotides (ddNTP) that are incapable of forming the next DNA bond in an elongation reaction. When incorporated into a synthesizing DNA strand, a ddNTP causes the strand elongation to stop. Labeling each of the 4 dideoxynucleotides with a different chromogen results, when the PCR is complete, in a reaction mix that contains a population of PCR fragments of different lengths, each terminating in a fluorescent dye-containing dideoxynucleotide, the specific dye corresponding to the final base on that fragment. The reaction is then run on a polyacrylamide electrophoresis gel in a sequencer, so that the fragments separate according to size, and as they run past a laser detector at the bottom of the gel, the emission wavelength (and hence identity of the terminal nucleic acid) of each fragment is detected.

instance, the presence of "dystrophic" features within muscle biopsies, such as large hypertrophied myofibers and increased connective and fatty tissues, characterized dystrophies, whereas congenital myopathies were categorized as relatively nonprogressive early-onset disorders with specific, nondystrophic pathologic features. Furthermore, congenital muscular dystrophies were so termed because of the dystrophic features on muscle histochemical studies and their frequent presence in infancy. However, some dystrophies do not have dystrophic features on muscle biopsies

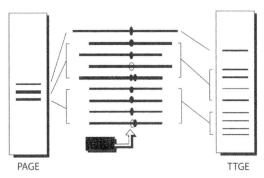

Fig. 6. Detection of new mutants. For gene alleles with similar polyacrylamide gel electrophoresis (PAGE) pattern, differing at a single base pair, denaturing produces 4 distinct single-stranded DNA sequences, and renaturing results in the random combination of these strands into the 2 original double-stranded segments ("homoduplexes") and 2 other double-stranded segments that differ at one base pair ("heteroduplexes"), and thus have a different denaturing profile in the temporal temperature gradient gel electrophoresis (TTGE).

(eg, some LGMDs, and myotonic dystrophy types 1 and 2), congenital myopathies may have adult onset (eg, nemaline myopathy) and progression, and distal myopathies may also have proximal weakness and be classified as LGMDs (dysferlin mutations).

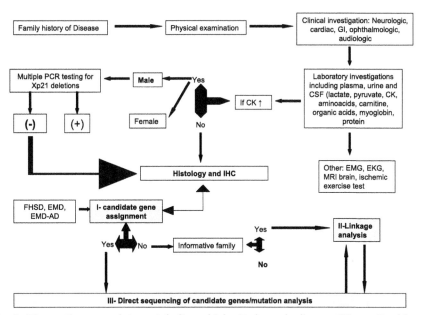

Fig. 7. Diagnostic approach to metabolic and inherited muscle disease. CK, creatine kinase; CSF, cerebrospinal fluid; EKG, electrocardiogram; EMD, Emery-Dreifuss muscular dystrophy; EMD-AD, Emery-Dreifuss muscular dystrophy autosomal dominant; EMG, electromyogram; FSHD, fascioscapulohumeral muscular dystrophy; IHC, immunohistochemistry; MRI, magnetic resonance imaging; P-MRS, phosphorous magnetic resonance spectroscopy.

Dystrophinopathies

The muscular dystrophies known as dystrophinopathies are classically characterized by 3 main clinical syndromes: Duchenne muscular dystrophy (DMD), Becker muscular dystrophy (BMD), and X-linked dilated cardiomyopathy. Clinically some dystrophin mutations can produce syndromes that are mistaken for other dystrophies, including LGMD[20] and facioscapulohumeral muscular dystrophy.[21]

The dystrophin gene is one of the largest known human genes. It contains 79 exons and its total size is around 2.4 million base pairs, approximately one-thousandth of the entire genome sequence. Therefore, testing for mutations is particularly complex. Roughly 60% of patients with DMD have large deletions of one or more exons, 35% have small or point mutations, and 5% have large duplications or chromosomal rearrangements.[22–26] Most large deletions are detected by RFLP analysis.[27] Because most deletions tend to occur in the same exons, called hot spots, PCR amplification and sequencing of limited numbers of exons is a suitable efficient technique and is able to detect almost all large deletions.[28] The most difficult task is detection of small mutations, which have to be detected by sequencing of multiple exons.[29] Denaturing techniques (single-strand conformation polymorphism, DGGE) detect 90% to 100% of mutations, though they will also detect other sequence variations not considered mutants, and require further analyses, usually sequencing, to determine whether the variation is a benign polymorphism or mutation.[18,30] Protein methods and muscle immunohistochemistry with antibodies directed against dystrophin may show absence of muscle dystrophin in DMD males and mosaic patterns in female carriers; however, genetic testing is more accurate.[31]

Limb girdle muscular dystrophies

Clinically characterized by predominant involvement of proximal arm and leg muscles, with type I being autosomal dominant and type II autosomal recessive, usually the LGMD phenotypes are not distinctive enough to allow for the use of DNA diagnostic testing as a first step.[32] However, particular mutations may present with distinctive features, such as with dysferlin (very high serum creatine kinase [CK]; prominent calf atrophy and weakness), caveolin-3 (coexisting rippling muscle disease),[33] lamin A/C (early elbow flexion and ankle plantar flexion contractures, cardiac conduction defects),[34] and calpain-3 (prominent scapular winging, weakness of shoulder adduction and elbow flexion, contractures, and severe posterior thigh involvement).[35] At present, the molecular diagnosis of most LGMDs is based on protein analysis from muscle biopsies with immunohistochemistry or Western blot, sometimes followed up with DNA testing. However, immunohistochemistry results must be interpreted cautiously, as a genetically based reduction in one sarcolemmal protein may result in secondary reduction in several other proteins and therefore confound interpretation.[36] For patients with a family history suggesting an autosomal-dominant limb girdle myopathy, lamin A/C mutations in blood specimens should be sought prior to muscle biopsy. By contrast, patients with a family history suggestive of autosomal-recessive inheritance might have sequential blood genetic testing for dysferlin (by Western blot), calpain-3, and fukutin-related protein, and only undergo muscle biopsy if these are negative (**Table 2**).

Myotonic dystrophies

Myotonic dystrophy is the second most common muscular dystrophy and is characterized by distal weakness, clinical myotonia, and multisystemic compromise including diabetes, cardiac conduction defects, and cataracts. Two different types have been described: type 1 results from CTG expansions in the DMPK gene[37] and

Table 2
Limb girdle muscular dystrophies

Disease	Gene	Cases	Testing Availability
LGMD1A	Myotilin	2 families	N/A
LGMD1B	Lamin A/C	Global	Sequencing all exons
LGMD1C	Caveolin-3	Global	N/A
LGMD1D	Unknown	2 families	N/A
LGMD1E	Unknown	2 families	N/A
LGMD1F	Unknown	1 family	N/A
LGMD2A	Calpin-3	Global	Sequencing all exons
LGMD2B	Dysferlin	Global	Western blot
LGMD2C	γ-Sarcoglycan	Global	Sequencing all exons
LGMD2D	α-Sarcoglycan	Global	Sequencing all exons
LGMD2E	β-Sarcoglycan	Global	Sequencing all exons
LGMD2F	δ-Sarcoglycan	Brazil	Denaturing DNA
LGMD2 G	Telethonin	3 families	N/A
LGMD2H	TRIM32	Inbred populations	N/A
LGMD2I	Fukutin-related protein	Global	Sequencing all exons
LGMD2J[a]	Titin	12 in Finland	N/A

Abbreviation: N/A, not available.
 [a] Autosomal dominant muscular dystrophy.

type 2 results from CTG expansions in the ZNF9 gene.[38] Both types have a similar phenotype.[39] Similarly, both mutations produce aberrant RNA transcripts, interfering with the processing of multiple other transcripts, for example, expression of chlorine channels and/or insulin receptors affecting multiple systems.[40,41] Molecular testing of type 1 is highly beneficial and is based on the evaluation of expanded repeats, changing the size of an intron.[42] A form of 35 repeats or fewer is considered normal; from 35 to 49 repeats is recognized as permutation, and is generally discovered in asymptomatic parents of symptomatic offspring whose repeat size has expanded to more than 50 alleles. Severity of disease is associated with increased repeat sizes.[43] Maternally transmitted alleles tend to present with severe phenotypes and increase size repeats more than the paternally transmitted counterpart.[44] By contrast, maternally transmitted severe congenital forms have not been identified in type 2, and there is no a clear correlation between large repeat size and severity as observed in molecular testing.[45]

Facioscapulohumeral muscular dystrophy
FSHD is a DNA disorder; however, it affects a region near the telomere of chromosome 4, with nonactive transcription regions.[46] Its mechanism is unknown. Normally this region contains 12 to 100 repeats, each one of 3.3 kb called the D4Z4. Chromosome 10 contains a highly homologous region that can result in homologous recombination and translocation with this chromosome 4 region, resulting in increased size in the chromosome 4.[47] Molecular diagnosis is based on RFLP techniques using double restriction enzyme digestion, which produces DNA fragments less than 35 kb in size and specific probes that are able to bind to chromosome 4 sequences and not to chromosome 10.[48] A different mechanism affecting the same DNA region in chromosome 4 has been described, which is associated with hypomethylation (epigenetics) of DNA

sequences and the same phenotype.[3] Three to five percent of FSHD cases do not have detectable mutations or epigenetic phenomena.[3]

Oculopharyngeal muscular dystrophy (OPMD)

Oculopharyngeal muscular dystrophy (OPMD) results from GCG triplet insertion in one allele for the polyadenylate binding protein 2 gene (PABP2).[49–51] The normal number of repeats is 6/6 (allele/allele). A combination 6/7 results in normal phenotype, but 7/7 is associated with autosomal-recessive pattern and 6/≥8 is autosomal dominant.[52] Genetic testing for OPMD is highly accurate (≈ 99%) and is performed by amplification and sequencing of the first exon of this gene.[53]

Emery-Dreifuss muscular dystrophies

Emery-Dreifuss muscular dystrophies (EMD) are the result of mutations in the emerin of lamin A/C (LMNA) gene, and clinically are characterized by myopathy with contractures and severe cardiac conduction defects.[54,55] These genes code for nuclear envelope proteins.[56] Molecular diagnosis is based on sequencing of X-linked emerin and LMNA. LMNA mutations are associated with different clinical phenotypes including autosomal-dominant EMD,[34] autosomal-recessive EMD,[57] LGMD 1B,[58] dilated cardiomyopathy with conduction defects,[59] familial lipodystrophy,[60] the premature aging syndrome progeria,[61] and inherited axonal neuropathy CMT2B1 or CMT4.[62]

Nondystrophic inherited myopathies with specific ultrastructural abnormalities

These disorders are defined by specific pathologic features, found in subcellular structures such as nemaline rods, central or multiple small cores, fibrillar Z-disc inclusions, and vacuolar inclusions. The disorders are included in this review because some of them can have progressive courses, with adolescent and even late adult onset. Classically these disorders are caused by abnormal accumulation of proteins.[63] For instance, nemaline myopathies result from point mutations in 5 different thin filament genes: ACTA1 (α-actin), TPM3 (α-tropomyosin), TPM2 (β-tropomyosin), NEB (nebulin), and TNNT1 (troponin T1). Clinical testing is available for ACTA1 mutations, accounting for 15% of patients with nemaline myopathy.[64,65]

Cores are identified as areas of myofibers with decreased oxidative enzyme activity, resulting from mutations of ryanodine receptor (RYR1)[66] and selenoprotein N1 (SEPN1).[67–69] Molecular genetic testing is clinically available for RYR1 mutations,[70] the major cause of malignant hyperthermia—especially in patients with anesthetic risk and muscle biopsy abnormalities consistent with central or multiple cores.

Myofibrillar myopathies (MFM) or desmin-related myopathies are characterized histologically by the accumulation of Z-disc fibrillar material. Ninety-five percent of patients in a series of 63 had onset after the age of 20 years.[63] Patients present clinically with proximal and distal weakness, and variable coexisting cardiomyopathy is common.[71] MFM are considered a group of genetically heterogeneous disorders, with mutations in α-B crystallin,[72] desmin,[73] myotilin,[74] and selenoprotein N.[75] The only one of these with a commercially available genetic test is selenoprotein N.

Nondystrophic myotonic disorders and periodic paralysis (channelopathies)

These conditions are the result of mutation in ion channels that clinically are manifested by transient hyperexcitability (myotonia), hypoexcitability (paralysis), or both.[76,77] Nondystrophic myotonias can affect the chloride channel gene CLCN1, encoding the ClC-1 protein (the same gene whose transcription is disrupted by the mutant RNA transcripts of myotonic dystrophy); they can have a dominant or recessive character.[78] Sodium channel subunit gene SCN4A mutations have a variable spectrum of phenotypes, including paramyotonia congenita,[79] potassium-aggravated myotonia,[80] and hyperkalemic[79] or hypokalemic periodic paralysis.[81]

Similarly, mutations in the calcium channel gene CACN1AS cause hypokalemic periodic paralysis,[82] in contrast to mutations in the potassium channel gene KCNJ2 or Andersen-Tawil syndrome that produce hypo-, normo-, or hyperkalemic periodic paralysis associated with characteristic facial features and long QT interval.[83,84]

Clinical investigations first should rule out myotonic dystrophies in patients with myotonia without paralysis or marked worsening in the cold.[76] CLCN1 mutations and Thomsen disease have specific genetic tests commercially available. On the contrary, patients with myotonia that increases during exercise and gets worse in the cold (paradoxic myotonia) and/or hyperkalemia periodic paralysis should be tested for SCN4A mutations, but if the myotonia is exacerbated only by cold and not by exercise, DMPK and ZNF9 testing is suggested. Patients with characteristic facial features and/or long QT interval should have KCNJ2 testing.

Mitochondrial myopathies

Mitochondrial disorders are increasingly being diagnosed, especially among patients with multiple, seemingly unrelated, neuromuscular and multisystem disorders. The genetics of these disorders are complex, because mutations can be located in the nuclear or mitochondrial genomes (mtDNA). Clinical syndromes are well defined and their associations with specific mutations are described, yet the genotype-phenotype correlation is not consistent, and many patients do not fit within any defined syndrome or have rare novel mutations. Another contributory factor is that mutant and wild-type mtDNA coexist (heteroplasmy), resulting in different degrees of syndrome severity, although homoplasmic mtDNA mutations also are known.

Aminoglycoside-induced or nonsyndromic deafness

These phenotypes have been reported as being associated with A1555 G, a point mutation in the mtDNA12S ribosomal RNA gene. However, 13 different mtDNA variants have been associated with deafness.[85]

Cyclic vomiting syndrome

Cyclic vomiting syndrome is characterized by stereotypical episodes of nausea, vomiting, and lethargy; with no clinical symptoms during episodes, it is considered a migraine variant. A large mtDNA rearrangement was found in one case.[86]

Kearns-Sayre syndrome

Kearns-Sayre syndrome (KSS) is defined as chronic progressive external ophthalmoplegia, atypical retinitis pigmentosa, proximal muscle weakness, with onset before age 20 years and one of the following: cardiac conduction defects, cerebellar ataxia or cerebrospinal fluid protein greater than 100 mg/dL. KSS is often caused by a single large 5-kb mtDNA deletion; however, additional possibilities include deletion/duplications and mtDNA point mutations including A3243 G.[87] At the level of the genome this syndrome is associated with mutations in adenine nucleotide translocator-1 (ANT1), Twinkle (a putative mtDNA helicase), and γ-polymerase (POLG).[88]

Leigh disease or subacute necrotizing encephalopathy

Leigh disease presents classically with cranial nerve abnormalities, respiratory dysfunction, and ataxia with hyperintense signals on T2-weighted images in the basal ganglia, cerebellum, or brain stem. Age of onset is from infancy to early childhood, with progressive course and high mortality. Genetically it is a heterogeneous disorder with very high mutant loads of the T8993 G/C mtDNA mutation (usually >95%); or nuclear DNA related to complex I deficiency (including NDUFV1 mutations), complex IV deficiency (including SURF1 mutations), and pyruvate dehydrogenase complex deficiency.[87]

Leber hereditary optic neuropathy
Characterized by rapid central visual loss in adolescents or young adults, this syndrome might be associated with dystonia. Leber hereditary optic neuropathy (LHON) is usually caused by homoplasmic mtDNA mutations, the most common being G11778A, G3460A, and T14484C.[87]

Mitochondrial encephalopathy, lactic acidosis, and stroke-like episodes
As described by its name, Mitochondrial encephalopathy, lactic acidosis, and stroke-like episodes (MELAS) is characterized by stroke-like episodes, potentially reversible, with onset between age 5 and 15 years though it can occur any time between infancy and adulthood, and lactic acidosis. Heteroplasmic in nature affecting mtDNA, MELAS mutations can compromise transfer RNA genes for leucine (A3243 G); however, other mutations have been described, such as T3217C or large rearrangements of mtDNA, and even nuclear DNA.[89,90]

Myoclonic epilepsy and ragged-red fiber disease
Myoclonic epilepsy and ragged-red fiber disease (MERRF) presents with progressive epilepsy, dementia, and symmetric lipomatosis, with onset in late childhood or adulthood. This syndrome has been associated with heteroplasmic point mutations of tRNA lysine (A8344 G).[91]

Usually mtDNA mutations can be diagnosed by multiple simultaneous PCR reactions that amplify the regions containing the common point mutations responsible for MELAS (A3243 G, T3271C), MERRF (A8344 G, T8356C), Leigh disease (T8993C, T8993 G), and LHON (G11778A, G3460A, T14484C and G14459A).[92] However, the molecular testing is not limited to this methodology and, in general, all the molecular techniques including sequencing have been used to detect significant mutations associated with mitochondrial disorders.[93,94] Testing for several of these disorders is typically done through muscle biopsy as well as measurements of respiratory enzyme activities. These measurements are technically challenging, with important pitfalls.[95–97]

FUTURE PERSPECTIVES

Within the last two decades the application of molecular genetic strategies has led to a delineation of subgroups of clinically indistinguishable neuromuscular disorders and has disclosed marked disease overlap. The expanding number of molecular defined NMDs requires new strategies to classify overlapping and clinically indistinguishable phenotypes. The objective of the science community in this field is to develop an economical molecular screening set for the most frequent neuromuscular disorders and to show its successful use for the detection of specific mutations. This method should be universally applicable and capable of extension to other diseases with overlapping phenotypes, such as distal myopathies, hereditary neuropathies, or the large groups of inherited hypertrophic and dilated cardiomyopathies.

REFERENCES

1. Flanagan SE, Patch AM, Ellard S. Using SIFT and PolyPhen to predict loss-of-function and gain-of-function mutations. Genet Test Mol Biomarkers 2010;14(4): 533–7.
2. Hackman P, Vihola A, Haravuori H, et al. Tibial muscular dystrophy is a titinopathy caused by mutations in TTN, the gene encoding the giant skeletal-muscle protein titin. Am J Hum Genet 2002;71:492–500.

3. van Overveld PG, Lemmers RJ, Sandkuijl LA, et al. Hypomethylation of D4Z4 in 4q-linked and non-4q-linked facioscapulohumeral muscular dystrophy. Nat Genet 2003;35:315–7.
4. Demir E, Sabatelli P, Allamand V, et al. Mutations in COL6A3 cause severe and mild phenotypes of Ullrich congenital muscular dystrophy. Am J Hum Genet 2002;70:1446–58.
5. Taylor RW, McDonnell MT, Blakely EL, et al. Genotypes from patients indicate no paternal mitochondrial DNA contribution. Ann Neurol 2003;54:521–4.
6. Miller FJ, Rosenfeldt FL, Zhang C, et al. Precise determination of mitochondrial DNA copy number in human skeletal and cardiac muscle by a PCR-based assay: lack of change of copy number with age. Nucleic Acids Res 2003;31:e61.
7. DiMauro S, Schon EA. Mitochondrial DNA mutations in human disease. Am J Med Genet 2001;106:18–26.
8. DiMauro S, Bonilla E, Davidson M, et al. Mitochondria in neuromuscular disorders. Biochim Biophys Acta 1998;1366(1/2):199–210.
9. Wong LJ, Lam CW. Alternative, noninvasive tissues for quantitative screening of mutant mitochondrial DNA. Clin Chem 1997;43(7):1241–3.
10. Deshpande A, Gans J, Graves SW, et al. A rapid multiplex assay for nucleic acid-based diagnostics. J Microbiol Methods 2010;80(2):155–63.
11. Nollau P, Wagener C. Methods for detection of point mutations: performance and quality assessment. IFCC Scientific Division, Committee on Molecular Biology Techniques. Clin Chem 1997;43(7):1114–28.
12. Cannizzaro LA, Shi G. Fluorescent in situ hybridization (FISH) for DNA probes in the interphase and metaphase stages of the cell cycle. Methods Mol Biol 1997; 75:313–22.
13. Wong LJ, Senadheera D. Direct detection of multiple point mutations in mitochondrial DNA. Clin Chem 1997;43(10):1857–61.
14. Randhawa J, Easton A. Demystified DNA nucleotide sequencing. Mol Pathol 1999;52:117–24.
15. Shendure J, Mitra RD, Varma C, et al. Advanced sequencing technologies: methods and goals. Nat Rev Genet 2004;5:335–44.
16. Fodde R, Losekoot M. Mutation detection by denaturing gradient gel electrophoresis (DGGE). Hum Mutat 1994;3:83–94.
17. Hoffman EP, Brown KJ, Eccleston E. New molecular research technologies in the study of muscle disease. Curr Opin Rheumatol 2003;15:698–707.
18. Dolinsky LC, de Moura-Neto RS, Falcao-Conceicao DN. DGGE analysis as a tool to identify point mutations, de novo mutations and carriers of the dystrophin gene. Neuromuscul Disord 2002;12:845–8.
19. Hofstra RM, Mulder IM, Vossen R, et al. DGGE-based whole-gene mutation scanning of the dystrophin gene in Duchenne and Becker muscular dystrophy patients. Hum Mutat 2004;23:57–66.
20. Beyenburg S, Zierz S, Arahata K, et al. Abnormal dystrophin expression in patients with limb girdle syndromes. J Neurol 1994;241:210–7.
21. Yamanaka G, Goto K, Ishihara T, et al. FSHD-like patients without 4q35 deletion. J Neurol Sci 2004;219:89–93.
22. Baumbach LL, Chamberlain JS, Ward PA, et al. Molecular and clinical correlations of deletions leading to Duchenne and Becker muscular dystrophies. Neurology 1989;39:465–74.
23. Den Dunnen JT, Grootscholten PM, Bakker E, et al. Topography of the Duchenne muscular dystrophy (DMD) gene: FIGE and cDNA analysis of 194 cases reveals 115 deletions and 13 duplications. Am J Hum Genet 1989;45:835–47.

24. Ikezawa M, Minami N, Takahashi M, et al. Dystrophin gene analysis on 130 patients with Duchenne muscular dystrophy with a special reference to muscle mRNA analysis. Brain Dev 1998;20:165–8.

25. Niemann-Seyde S, Slomski R, Rininsland F, et al. Molecular genetic analysis of 67 patients with Duchenne/Becker muscular dystrophy. Hum Genet 1992;90: 65–70.

26. White S, Kalf M, Liu Q, et al. Comprehensive detection of genomic duplications and deletions in the DMD gene, by use of multiplex amplifiable probe hybridization. Am J Hum Genet 2002;71:365–74.

27. Darras BT, Koenig M, Kunkel, et al. Direct method for prenatal diagnosis and carrier detection in Duchenne/Becker muscular dystrophy using the entire dystrophin cDNA. Am J Med Genet 1988;29:713–26.

28. Beggs AH, Koenig M, Boyce FM, et al. Detection of 98% of DMD/BMD gene deletions by polymerase chain reaction. Hum Genet 1990;86:45–8.

29. Flanigan KM, von Niederhausern A, Dunn DM, et al. Rapid direct sequence analysis of the dystrophin gene. Am J Hum Genet 2003;72:931–9.

30. Mendell JR, Buzin CH, Feng J, et al. Diagnosis of Duchenne dystrophy by enhanced detection of small mutations. Neurology 2001;57:645–50.

31. Hoffman EP, Fischbeck KH, Brown RH, et al. Characterization of dystrophin in muscle biopsy specimens from patients with Duchenne's or Becker's muscular dystrophy. N Engl J Med 1988;318:1363–8.

32. van der Kooi AJ, Barth PG, Busch HF, et al. The clinical spectrum of limb girdle muscular dystrophy. A survey in The Netherlands. Brain 1996;119(Pt 5):1471–80.

33. Fee DB, So YT, Barraza C, et al. Phenotypic variability associated with Arg26Gln mutation in caveolin3. Muscle Nerve 2004;30:375–8.

34. Bonne G, Mercuri E, Muchir A, et al. Clinical and molecular genetic spectrum of autosomal dominant Emery-Dreifuss muscular dystrophy due to mutations of the lamin A/C gene. Ann Neurol 2000;48:170–80.

35. Pollitt C, Anderson LVB, Pogue R, et al. The phenotype of calpainopathy: diagnosis based on a multidisciplinary approach. Neuromuscul Disord 2001;11: 287–96.

36. Cohn RD, Campbell KP. Molecular basis of muscular dystrophies. Muscle Nerve 2000;23:1456–71.

37. Brook JD, McCurrach ME, Harley HG, et al. Molecular basis of myotonic dystrophy: expansion of a trinucleotide (CTG) repeat at the 3 end of a transcript encoding a protein kinase family member. Cell 1992;68:799–808.

38. Udd B, Meola G, Krahe R, et al. Report of the 115th ENMC workshop: DM2/PROMM and other myotonic dystrophies. 3rd workshop, 14–16 February 2003, Naarden, The Netherlands. Neuromuscul Disord 2003;13:589–96.

39. Thornton CA, Griggs RC, Moxley RT III. Myotonic dystrophy with no trinucleotide repeat expansion. Ann Neurol 1994;35:269–72.

40. Ranum LP, Day JW. Myotonic dystrophy: RNA pathogenesis comes into focus. Am J Hum Genet 2004;74:793–804.

41. Savkur RS, Philips AV, Cooper TA, et al. Insulin receptor splicing alteration in myotonic dystrophy type 2. Am J Hum Genet 2004;74:1309–13.

42. International Myotonic Dystrophy Consortium (IDMC). New nomenclature and DNA testing guidelines for myotonic dystrophy type 1 (DM1). Neurology 2000; 54:1218–21.

43. Harley HG, Rundle SA, MacMillan JC, et al. Size of the unstable CTG repeat sequence in relation to phenotype and parental transmission in myotonic dystrophy. Am J Hum Genet 1993;52:1164–74.

44. Lavedan C, Hofmann-Radvanyi H, Shelbourne P, et al. Myotonic dystrophy: size-and sex-dependent dynamics of CTG meiotic instability, and somatic mosaicism. Am J Hum Genet 1993;52:875–83.
45. Day JW, Ricker K, Jacobsen JF, et al. Myotonic dystrophy type 2: molecular, diagnostic and clinical spectrum. Neurology 2003;60:657–64.
46. Sarfarazi M, Wijmenga C, Upadhyaya M, et al. Regional mapping of facioscapulohumeral muscular dystrophy gene on 4q35: combined analysis of an international consortium. Am J Hum Genet 1992;51:396–403.
47. van Overveld PG, Lemmers RJFL, Deidda G, et al. Interchromosomal repeat array interactions between chromosomes 4 and 10: a model for subtelomeric plasticity. Hum Mol Genet 2000;9:2879–84.
48. Upadhyaya M, Maynard J, Rogers MT, et al. Improved molecular diagnosis of facioscapulohumeral muscular dystrophy (FSHD): validation of the differential double digestion for FSHD. J Med Genet 1997;34:476–9.
49. Brais B, Bouchard JP, Xie YG, et al. Short GCG expansions in the PABP2 gene cause oculopharyngeal muscular dystrophy. Nat Genet 1998;18:164–7.
50. Hill ME, Creed GA, McMullan TF, et al. Oculopharyngeal muscular dystrophy: phenotypic and genotypic studies in a UK population. Brain 2001;124:522–6.
51. Mirabella M, Silvestri G, de Rosa G, et al. GCG genetic expansions in Italian patients with oculopharyngeal muscular dystrophy. Neurology 2000;54:608–14.
52. Brais B. Oculopharyngeal muscular dystrophy: a late-onset polyalanine disease. Cytogenet Genome Res 2003;100:252–60.
53. van der Sluijs BM, van Engelen BG, Hoefsloot LH. Oculopharyngeal muscular dystrophy (OPMD) due to a small duplication in the PABPN1 gene. Hum Mutat 2003;21:553.
54. Bione S, Maestrini E, Rivella S, et al. Identification of a novel X-linked gene responsible for Emery-Dreifuss muscular dystrophy. Nat Genet 1994;8:323–7.
55. Bonne G, Di Barletta MR, Varnous S, et al. Mutations in the gene encoding lamin A/C cause autosomal dominant Emery-Dreifuss muscular dystrophy. Nat Genet 1999;21:285–8.
56. Wilson KL. The nuclear envelope, muscular dystrophy and gene expression. Trends Cell Biol 2000;10:125–9.
57. Raffaele Di Barletta M, Ricci E, Galluzzi G, et al. Different mutations in the LMNA gene cause autosomal dominant and autosomal recessive Emery-Dreifuss muscular dystrophy. Am J Hum Genet 2000;66:1407–12.
58. Muchir A, Bonne G, van der Kooi AJ, et al. Identification of mutations in the gene encoding lamins A/C in autosomal dominant limb girdle muscular dystrophy with atrioventricular conduction disturbances (LGMD1B). Hum Mol Genet 2000;9: 1453–9.
59. Fatkin D, MacRae C, Sasaki T, et al. Missense mutations in the rod domain of the lamin A/C gene as causes of dilated cardiomyopathy and conduction-system disease. N Engl J Med 1999;341:1715–24.
60. Cao H, Hegele RA. Nuclear lamin A/C R482Q mutation in Canadian kindreds with Dunnigan-type familial partial lipodystrophy. Hum Mol Genet 2000;9:109–12.
61. Eriksson M, Brown WT, Gordon LB, et al. Recurrent de novo point mutations in lamin A cause Hutchinson-Gilford progeria syndrome. Nature 2003;423: 293–8.
62. De Sandre-Giovannoli A, Chaouch M, Kozlov S, et al. Homozygous defects in LMNA, encoding lamin A/C nuclear-envelope proteins, cause autosomal recessive axonal neuropathy in human (Charcot- Marie-Tooth disorder type 2) and mouse. Am J Hum Genet 2002;70:726–36.

63. Goebel HH. Congenital myopathies at their molecular dawning. Muscle Nerve 2003;27:527–48.
64. Wallgren-Pettersson C, Pelin K, Nowak KJ, et al. Genotype-phenotype correlations in nemaline myopathy caused by mutations in the genes for nebulin and skeletal muscle alpha-actin. Neuromuscul Disord 2004;14:461–70.
65. Sanoudou D, Beggs AH. Clinical and genetic heterogeneity in nemaline myopathy—a disease of skeletal muscle thin filaments. Trends Mol Med 2001;7:362–8.
66. Ryan MM, Schnell C, Strickland CD, et al. Nemaline myopathy: a clinical study of 143 cases. Ann Neurol 2001;50:312–20.
67. Zhang Y, Chen HS, Khanna VK, et al. A mutation in the human ryanodine receptor gene associated with central core disease. Nat Genet 1993;5:46–50.
68. Ferreiro A, Quijano-Roy S, Pichereau C, et al. Mutations of the selenoprotein N gene, which is implicated in rigid spine muscular dystrophy, cause the classical phenotype of multiminicore disease: reassessing the nosology of early-onset myopathies. Am J Hum Genet 2002;71:739–49.
69. Moghadaszadeh B, Petit N, Jaillard C, et al. Mutations in SEPN1 cause congenital muscular dystrophy with spinal rigidity and restrictive respiratory syndrome. Nat Genet 2001;29:17–8.
70. Kraev N, Loke JC, Kraev A, et al. Protocol for the sequence analysis of ryanodine receptor subtype 1 gene transcripts from human leukocytes. Anesthesiology 2003;99:289–96.
71. Selcen D, Ohno K, Engel AG. Myofibrillar myopathy: clinical, morphological and genetic studies in 63 patients. Brain 2004;127:439–51.
72. Engel AG. Myofibrillar myopathy. Ann Neurol 1999;46:681–3.
73. Vicart P, Caron A, Guicheney P, et al. A missense mutation in the alphaB-crystallin chaperone gene causes a desmin-related myopathy. Nat Genet 1998;20:92–5.
74. Dalakas MC, Park KY, Semino-Mora C, et al. Desmin myopathy, a skeletal myopathy with cardiomyopathy caused by mutations in the desmin gene. N Engl J Med 2000;342:770–80.
75. Selcen D, Engel AG. Mutations in myotilin cause myofibrillar myopathy. Neurology 2004;62:1363–71.
76. Lehmann-Horn F, Rudel R, Jurkat-Rott K. Nondystrophic myotonias and periodic paralysis. In: Engel AG, Franzini- Armstrong C, editors. Myology. 3rd edition. New York: McGraw- Hill; 2004. p. 1257–300.
77. Koch MC, Steinmeyer K, Lorenz C, et al. The skeletal muscle chloride channel in dominant and recessive human myotonia. Science 1992;257:797–800.
78. Pusch M. Myotonia caused by mutations in the muscle chloride channel gene CLCN1. Hum Mutat 2002;19:423–34.
79. Ebers GC, George AL, Barchi RL, et al. Paramyotonia congenita and hyperkalemic periodic paralysis are linked to the adult muscle sodium channel gene. Ann Neurol 1991;30:810–6.
80. Heine R, Pika U, Lehmann-Horn F. A novel SCN4A mutation causing myotonia aggravated by cold and potassium. Hum Mol Genet 1993;2:1349–53.
81. Bulman DE, Scoggan KA, van Oene MD, et al. A novel sodium channel mutation in a family with hypokalemic periodic paralysis. Neurology 1999;53:1932–6.
82. Ptacek LJ, Tawil R, Griggs RC, et al. Dihydropyridine receptor mutations cause hypokalemic periodic paralysis. Cell 1994;77:863–8.
83. Plaster NM, Tawil R, Tristani-Firouzi M, et al. Mutations in Kir2.1 cause the developmental and episodic electrical phenotypes of Andersen's syndrome. Cell 2001;105:511–9.

84. Kim JB, Chung KW. Novel de novo mutation in the KCNJ2 gene in a patient with Andersen-Tawil syndrome. Pediatr Neurol 2009;41(6):464–6.
85. Wallace DC, Ruiz-Pesini E, Mishmar D. mtDNA variation, climatic adaptation, degenerative diseases, and longevity. Cold Spring Harb Symp Quant Biol 2003;68:479–86.
86. Boles RG, Chun N, Senadheera D, et al. Cyclic vomiting syndrome and mitochondrial DNA mutations. Lancet 1997;350:1299–300.
87. Wallace DC, Lott MT, Brown MD, et al. Mitochondria and neuro-ophthalmologic diseases. In: Scriver CR, Beaudet AL, Sly WS, et al, editors. The metabolic & molecular bases of inherited disease. 8th edition. New York: McGraw-Hill; 2001. p. 2425–509.
88. Hirano M. Mitochondrial disorders due to mutations in the nuclear genome. In: Rosenberg RN, Prusiner SB, DiMauro S, et al, editors. The molecular and genetic basis of neurologic and psychiatric disease. 3rd edition. Boston: Butterworth-Heinemann; 2003. p. 197–204.
89. Shah NS, Mitchell WG, Boles RG. Mitochondrial disorders: a potentially under-recognized etiology of infantile spasms. J Child Neurol 2002;17:369–72.
90. Harrison TJ, Boles RG, Johnson DR, et al. Macular pattern retinal dystrophy, adult-onset diabetes, and deafness: a family study of A3243G mitochondrial heteroplasmy. Am J Ophthalmol 1997;124:217–21.
91. Shoffner JM. Oxidative phosphorylation diseases. In: Scriver CR, Beaudet AL, Sly WS, et al, editors. The metabolic and molecular bases of inherited disease. 8th edition. New York: McGraw-Hill; 2001. p. 2367–424.
92. Liang MH, Wong L-JC. Yield of mtDNA mutation analysis in 2000 patients. Am J Med Genet 1998;77:385–400.
93. DeMarchi JM, Richards CS, Fenwick RG, et al. A robotics-assisted procedure for large scale cystic fibrosis mutation analysis. Hum Mutat 1994;4:281–90.
94. van Den Bosch BJ, de Coo RF, Scholte HR, et al. Mutation analysis of the entire mitochondrial genome using denaturing high performance liquid chromatography. Nucleic Acids Res 2000;28:E89.
95. Chretien D, Slama A, Briere JJ, et al. Revisiting pitfalls, problems and tentative solutions for assaying mitochondrial respiratory chain complex III in human samples. Curr Med Chem 2004;11:233–9.
96. Janssen AJM, Smeitink JAM, van den Heuvel LP. Some practical aspects of providing a diagnostic service for respiratory chain defects. Ann Clin Biochem 2003;40:3–8.
97. Taylor RW, Schaefer AM, Barron MJ, et al. The diagnosis of mitochondrial muscle disease. Neuromuscul Disord 2004;14:237–45.

Essential Muscle Pathology for the Rheumatologist

Brent T. Harris, MD, PhD[a,b,*], Carrie A. Mohila, MD, PhD[c]

KEYWORDS

• Myopathy • Myositis • Muscle biopsy

INTRODUCTION TO MUSCLE BIOPSY AND BASIC HISTOPATHOLOGIC CHANGES IN SKELETAL MUSCLE

This review introduces/refreshes some basic histopathologic methods and findings of skeletal muscle biopsies with emphasis on those diseases commonly encountered in a rheumatologist's practice. The 3 general areas of myopathology discussed are metabolic myopathies, toxic myopathies, and inflammatory myopathies. Although there is considerable overlap in the patient populations with muscle-based illness for the rheumatologist and neurologist, the rheumatologist is more likely to encounter patients with these 3 classes of myopathy.

The authors, neuropathologists, hope to provide in this article what they think are some commonalities and disease-specific methods in their pathologic workup as well as a practical approach to the collaboration that pathologists undertake with their rheumatology colleagues to come to a working diagnosis. Neonatal, pediatric, dystrophic, and neuropathic myopathies are beyond the scope of this article. Also, much of the basic biochemistry, genetics, clinical presentations, and therapy for muscle diseases are more thoroughly covered in other disease-specific reviews.

Biopsy of the skeletal muscle is an important diagnostic study for many muscle diseases and in some cases is still the gold standard. However, this technique is often appropriately held in reserve to be done after a full noninvasive workup has been completed. Although not usually debilitating to patients, biopsy procedures can be

[a] Department of Pathology, Georgetown University Medical Center, Georgetown University, Building D, Room 207, 4000 Reservoir Road, NW, Washington, DC 20057, USA
[b] Department of Neurology, Georgetown University Medical Center, Georgetown University, Building D, Room 207, 4000 Reservoir Road, NW, Washington, DC 20057, USA
[c] Division of Neuropathology, Department of Pathology, University of Virginia Health System, Hospital Expansion Room 3069, 1215 Lee Street, PO Box 800214, Charlottesville, VA 22908, USA
* Corresponding author. Department of Neurology, Georgetown University Medical Center, Georgetown University, Building D, Room 207, 4000 Reservoir Road, NW, Washington, DC 20057.
E-mail address: BTH@Georgetown.edu

Rheum Dis Clin N Am 37 (2011) 289–308
doi:10.1016/j.rdc.2011.01.010
0889-857X/11/$ – see front matter © 2011 Elsevier Inc. All rights reserved.

painful and carry the standard risks of postsurgical infection and discomfort. Many of the cases that the surgical neuropathologist worked up in the last century by histologic methods are now diagnosed without a biopsy by molecular diagnostic laboratories using blood samples. However, many muscle diseases treated by rheumatologists still need some combination of histopathologic, biochemical, and genetic work up on the muscle tissue itself. Despite the diagnostic tools available today, the diverse and subtle clinical presentations of patients make muscle diseases some of the most challenging conditions to diagnose in medicine.

Biopsy Considerations

Several factors come into play when rheumatologists decide to pursue a muscle biopsy in the diagnostic workup. First, is the institution/practice set up to handle this kind of surgery and these complex specimens? The rheumatologist should talk to the pathologist before considering the biopsy. If they do not handle these specimens regularly, it is essential that the patient be referred to the nearest institution with a neuropathologist on staff to have the biopsy performed there. If this is not a possibility, the biopsy can be done remotely and the sample sent by courier (not mailed) on ice in a saline-moistened gauze wrap to the neuropathologist, provided the sample can be delivered within an hour or two maximum. However, this step is not optimal, and communication/coordination before the surgery with the on-site pathologist and the off-site neuropathologist is essential. Regardless of where the biopsy is done, liquid nitrogen should be available in the operating room (OR)/procedure room to rapidly freeze a portion of the muscle immediately at the time of resection. This flash frozen tissue is used for biochemical and genetic analyses, as indicated.

The next factor is who will do the biopsy. Different physicians in different institutions/practices perform this fairly minor surgery. With training, any physician can perform this surgery, and many rheumatologists and neurologists handle these cases for their patients, a real preference by the pathologists because rheumatologists and neurologists can generally be in better communication about what should be technically done with the specimens at the time of surgery and in conveying the findings. If the patient is referred for the biopsy to a general surgeon, there should be communication between the rheumatologist, the surgeon, and the pathologist to coordinate logistics. Which muscle to biopsy is an important consideration—a muscle that is clinically affected but not in end-stage should be chosen. Magnetic resonance imaging is gaining popularity to help distinguish muscle groups with inflammation[1]; however, clinical judgment is still needed. The surgeon should be in contact with the pathologist to discuss how many samples are needed for the case and to arrange for the liquid nitrogen to be on-hand in the OR. Having a pathology assistant or technician come to the OR to manage the specimens can be helpful.

Once the specimens are obtained, what tests need to be performed on them? The pathologist in most cases performs some standard processing and then works with the clinical team to come up with additional studies based on the clinical suspicions and initial histopathologic findings. Most muscle biopsy specimens have a portion fixed in buffered formalin for standard hematoxylin-eosin (H&E) histologic analysis, a portion fixed in glutaraldehyde for possible electron microscopic (EM) analysis, a portion frozen in a controlled manner for frozen section histochemical stainings, and one or more pieces flash frozen in liquid nitrogen for biochemical/genetic analyses. Specialized testing for many biochemical/genetic analyses often needs specimens to be sent out to one of a few reference laboratories that can perform the testing.

General Histopathology of Neuropathic, Myopathic, and Inflammatory Causes

Although the goal of the pathologist is to define as specifically as possible the pathologic diagnosis of the surgical specimen, with muscle biopsies, sometimes, the best one can do is categorizing them as most likely because of 1 of the following 3 causes: (1) myopathic in which the pathogenesis involves an intrinsic skeletal muscle disease that could be caused by genetic alterations, metabolic dysfunction, or toxic insult; (2) neuropathic (also called neurogenic), in which the observed muscle changes are caused by motor neuron injury/degeneration; or (3) inflammatory in which the change is caused by systemic immune system dysfunction or intrinsic muscle disease eliciting an inflammatory response. The cause of the disease dictates how the muscle will respond acutely and chronically and what will be the findings on histologic examination.

Neuropathic changes to muscle are brought about by deinnervation and sometimes reinnervation of myocytes by motor neurons. This change could occur with vasculitis that injures the motor neuron or a neurodegenerative process such as amyotrophic lateral sclerosis. The normal cross section of a myocyte is generally round or slightly polygonal, and there is minimal variation in fiber size in the tissue. Deinnervation causes myofibers to atrophy and have more sharp acute angles on cross section (**Fig. 1**A). Another common change in neuropathic myopathies is fiber type grouping into type I and type II fibers rather than the normal fairly even distribution of fibers or the so-called checkerboard pattern, which is highlighted best by ATPase histochemical stain on frozen section (see **Fig. 1**B). Finally, target fibers can be seen on frozen sections stained with NADH, which show clearing of the central portion of the myocyte.

Myopathic changes are more varied than those of neuropathic changes. There can also be marked variation in myofiber size and shape with both severe atrophy and hypertrophy of fibers, but usually, the fibers maintain more rounded contours. In long-standing processes, fibrosis is often seen between the individual myocytes. Degenerating and regenerating myofibers that take on a bluish color with H&E stain can often be seen in myopathic processes. Because these fibers are degenerating, lymphocytes and macrophages can be seen around and within the fiber as it breaks down, although infiltrates are usually minimal. Congenital myopathies and dystrophies that involve derangement of structural proteins of the cytoskeleton or extracellular matrix are examples in this category of myopathic change. Metabolic and toxic myopathies are also in this category and described in subsequent sections.

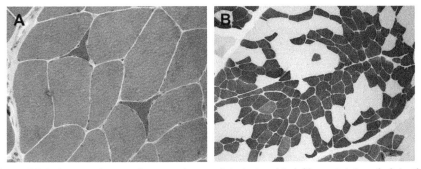

Fig. 1. (*A*) Deinnervation causing acutely angulated atrophied fibers staining dark in this case (esterase) (original magnification ×200). (*B*) Grouped atrophy showing dark (type I) and light (type II) fibers (ATPase) (original magnification ×40).

Inflammatory myopathic changes as a result of intrinsic muscle disease or systemic inflammatory conditions display variable types and amounts of immune cell infiltrates and myocyte injury. Some diseases smolder and display chronic inflammatory changes, whereas others run rampant through the affected muscle with acute inflammation and myocyte damage.

METABOLIC MYOPATHIES

Metabolic myopathies comprise a large group of maladies that span all age groups and have diverse causes that generally alter the intermediary metabolic biochemistry of myocytes. Many of these diseases can affect other tissues, especially those of the central nervous system. Diseases with a prominent muscle pathologic condition tend to have disruption in lipid or glycogen metabolism or mitochondrial functions such as oxidative phosphorylation. Defects in nearly every component of the lipid or carbohydrate metabolic pathways have been described in the literature.

Mitochondrial Myopathies

These disorders are the most common of the metabolic myopathies with highly variable severity affecting both young and old. Mutations or other genetic alterations in either mitochondrial or nuclear genes can lead to enzyme deficiencies and mitochondrial structural alterations that can be determined with biochemical testing and light and ultrastructural microscopy, respectively. Given the variable genes involved, the genetics is complex, and these diseases can be sporadic or familial following either Mendelian or non-Mendelian maternal transmission when mitochondrial gene alterations are involved.[2] With multiple organ involvement common, several syndromes such as Kearns-Sayre syndrome; Leigh syndrome; mitochondrial myopathy, encephalopathy, lactic acidosis, and strokelike episodes (MELAS); and myoclonic epilepsy, ragged red fibers (MERRF) have been recognized for sometime and the gene mutations involved have been identified more recently.

Several histologic hallmarks of mitochondrial myopathies (MMs) assist in making a preliminary diagnosis and are used in conjunction with the clinical picture and biochemical/genetic analyses to solidify a diagnosis. Mitochondria are numerous and diffusely arrayed within normal myocytes. In most MMs, ragged red fibers are readily seen and are so named, because on modified Gomori trichrome stain, the affected irregular myocytes stain reddish (**Fig. 2**A). The stain picks up accumulations

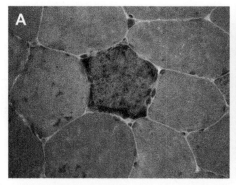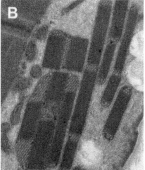

Fig. 2. Mitochondrial myopathy. (*A*) Ragged red fiber (Gomori trichrome stain, original magnification ×400). (*B*) Electron micrograph of paracrystalline mitochondrial inclusions (original magnification ×5000).

of mitochondria, often in a subsarcolemmal localization. Additional stains that can be useful in the workup of MM include NADH and succinate dehydrogenase, which show increased staining in aggregates; cytochrome c oxidase (COX), which does not stain in some MMs; and lipid stains such as oil red O, which highlight increased lipid deposition. The burden of ragged red fibers is highly variable, and sometimes they are not picked up on small biopsies. Conversely, rare ragged red fibers can be seen normally in elderly patients or in patients taking some drugs such as zidovudine (AZT).[3,4] So identification, although helpful, is not entirely sensitive or specific. Ultrastructural analysis by EM can be helpful. Alteration of sizes, shapes, and numbers of atypical mitochondria are found in affected fibers and suggest that the gene mutations involved could be altering the replication and structure of mitochondria in addition to key enzyme activities either directly or indirectly. Bizarre-appearing paracrystalline inclusions can sometimes be found within the mitochondria (see **Fig.** 2B).

Glycogenoses

Glycogen is the main storage molecule for glucose in the body and found primarily in liver and muscle tissue. With defects in the biosynthetic and breakdown pathways of glycogen metabolism, the storage and/or breakdown to glucose is diminished when needed for energy. Therefore, muscle cramping and fatigue or persistent muscle weakness are the prevailing presentations of glycogenoses (also called glycogen storage diseases [GSDs]). Some of the more common types of glycogenoses include McArdle disease (myophosphorylase deficiency, GSD type V), Pompe disease (acid maltase deficiency, GSD type II), and Tarui disease (phosphofructokinase deficiency, GSD type VII). Many other less-common glycogenoses are also recognized with nomenclatures based on genetics and discovery dates. To date, 11 glycogenoses associated with myopathy are known.[5]

A microscopic examination of muscle in glycogenoses can show very little pathology on H&E stain as in McArdle disease or can display abundant accumulation of glycogen in the so-called glycogen pools (**Fig. 3**) of other glycogenoses. Communicating with the pathologist the clinical suspicion for GSD is essential so that nonstandard staining for activity of enzymes such as myophosphorylase or phosphofructokinase can be added to the battery of stains or so that tissue can be analyzed biochemically for enzyme activity. Periodic acid–Schiff staining with and without diastase helps to highlight glycogen stores. EM can also delineate glycogen and show increased lysosomes with glycogen in diseases such as Pompe disease.

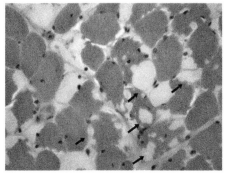

Fig. 3. Glycogen storage disease. Lightly stained pools of glycogen (*arrows*) (H&E, original magnification ×200).

Mutation analyses are available for most glycogenoses and can be performed on either lymphocytes or muscles.

Fatty Acid Oxidation Defects

Fatty acid oxidation metabolism myopathies are another common class of metabolic myopathies characterized by lipid accumulations within the muscle. These disorders are caused by defects in enzymes in free fatty acid beta oxidation that prevent the appropriate transport of lipids across the mitochondrial membrane for energy use. Carnitine, which is biosynthesized from amino acids, plays a major role in this transport process. Deficiencies of carnitine either systemically or specifically in the muscle can occur because of inherited mutations or can be drug-induced (valproate therapy).[5] Muscle biopsies often reveal vacuoles and increased lipid storage on oil red O staining. Carnitine palmityltransferase deficiencies of several types are also recognized often early in childhood with cramping and myoglobinuria, but can also manifest in adulthood. These patients generally do not show many histopathologic changes on biopsy and require genetic/biochemical enzyme analyses to make the diagnoses. Similarly, acyl-coenzyme A (CoA) dehydrogenase deficiencies show few, if any, histopathologic changes and must be screened for genetically/biochemically.

Myoadenylate Deaminase Deficiency

Myoadenylate deaminase converts AMP into ammonia and inosine monophosphate, which is important to driving ATP synthesis. The deficiency of this enzyme is common in the general population and often asymptomatic. However, increased stress and/or increased intolerance to exercise with cramping can occur in some affected individuals. Muscle biopsies show no abnormalities with commonly used stains. However, if myoadenylate deaminase histochemistry is performed, variable, but often complete, loss of staining will occur in these cases confirming the diagnosis.

IDIOPATHIC INFLAMMATORY MYOPATHIES

Inflammatory myopathies are classically divided into infectious and idiopathic (ie, noninfectious) etiologies. The idiopathic inflammatory myopathies (IIMs) are a heterogeneous group of rare disorders that include dermatomyositis (DM), polymyositis (PM), and sporadic inclusion body myositis (sIBM). The dominant clinical manifestation of the IIMs is skeletal muscle weakness. IIMs are distinguished from each other based on clinical signs and symptoms, laboratory and serologic tests, electromyography, and histopathologic findings. On muscle biopsy, all the 3 IIMs share the histologic feature of an inflammatory cell infiltrate. The pattern and composition of the infiltrate and identification of salient histologic features unique to each of the IIMs helps differentiate among them.[6,7] This section summarizes the main histopathologic findings that characterize the IIMs. The clinical features and underlying pathogenic mechanisms of IIMs are briefly discussed in this article but are extensively reviewed elsewhere.[8-11]

DM

The most common IIM is DM. DM is a multisystem disorder of adults and children that presents with muscle weakness, cutaneous disease, and systemic features. The skeletal muscle weakness is classically proximal, symmetric, and progressive over weeks to months. Cutaneous involvement of DM occurs early in the disease, even preceding muscle weakness,[12] and includes heliotrope rash and Gottron papules.[13] Heliotrope rash is a symmetric violaceous eruption of the periorbital skin that may be associated with scaling, desquamation, and/or massive periorbital edema. Gottron papules are elevated erythematous papules frequently with telangiectasia found over bony prominences, especially knuckles. Other cutaneous findings include photosensitivity, periungual telangiectasia, and poikiloderma of the anterior part of the neck and chest (V sign) and upper part of the back and shoulders (shawl sign). Systemic manifestations include arthralgias, dyspnea secondary to pulmonary disease, conduction defects and arrhythmias due to cardiac involvement, and dysphasia secondary to involvement of pharyngeal and/or upper esophageal skeletal muscles.[13,14] DM can also be seen in association with systemic sclerosis and mixed connective tissue disease.[14] Patients with DM also have an increased risk of various malignancies, including ovarian, gastrointestinal, pulmonary, and breast carcinomas and non-Hodgkin lymphoma.[15,16]

Laboratory studies reveal that serum creatine kinase (CK) levels can be normal or elevated (up to 50-fold).[17] Serologic testing often reveals the presence of myositis-associated autoantibodies (MAAs) and/or myositis-specific antibodies (MSAs).[18,19] MAAs are associated not only with myositis but also with various connective tissue disorders and include anti-U1-ribonucleoprotein, anti-Ro (SS-A), and anti-PM/scleroderma antibodies.[20] MSAs are primarily associated with myositis. Antibodies against histidyl-transfer RNA (tRNA)-synthetase (anti–Jo-1) are the most common MSAs and identify a clinical subgroup (anti-synthase syndrome) that combines myositis, interstitial lung disease, nonerosive arthritis, fever, and Raynaud phenomenon. Other MSAs include various anti–aminoacyl-tRNA synthetases, anti–Mi-2, and anti–signal recognition particle.

The myopathologic hallmark of DM is perifascicular myofiber atrophy characterized by abnormal small fibers at the periphery of muscle fascicles (ie, bundles of muscle fibers) **(Fig. 4**A). Myofibers adjacent to perimysial connective tissue are preferentially affected, whereas myofibers bordering other fascicles are less affected.[9] Perifascicular myofibers can also undergo necrosis, degeneration, and regeneration characterized by basophilic sarcoplasm and increased numbers of internalized myonuclei. Microinfarcts characterized by wedge-shaped areas of necrosis are rarely found.[6] Severely affected fibers can become vacuolated and may become partially reactive or nonreactive to histochemical stains (ghost fibers).[21] Myopathic changes are typically multifocal and can vary in severity in different regions of the same muscle biopsy. Histochemical stains for ATPase reveal that both type I and II fibers are affected. NADH activity is increased in the affected muscle fibers. Immunohistochemical stains

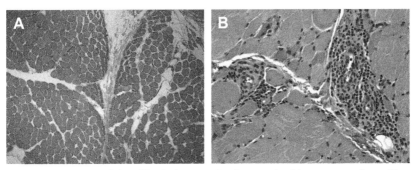

Fig. 4. Dermatomyositis. (*A*) Perifascicular atrophy characterized by many small myofibers at the periphery of muscle fascicles (original magnification ×40). (*B*) Inflammatory infiltrate located in the perivascular space composed primarily of B lymphocytes (H&E, original magnification ×100).

for major histocompatibility complex (MHC) class I reveals abnormal upregulation of MHC class I in the sarcolemma of perifascicular myofibers.[22]

DM is also characterized by an inflammatory infiltrate within the perimysium (ie, the connective tissue surrounding muscle fascicles) or in the perivascular space (see **Fig. 4**B). The inflammatory infiltrate is composed primarily of CD20+ B cells, macrophages, and CD4+ T cells and plasmacytoid dendritic cells.[23] The perimysial inflammatory infiltrate may focally extend into the endomysium at the periphery of fascicles, but invasion into individual myofibers is rarely seen. Intramuscular blood vessels may show vessel wall thickening, endothelial hyperplasia, vacuolization, and/or necrosis with loss of vessels in severe cases.[8] Lumens of residual capillaries are frequently dilated.[6] Decreased numbers of vessels can be detected with the lectin Ulex europaeus agglutinin I. Deposition of complement on the walls of intramuscular blood vessels can be detected with antibodies against C5b-9 complement membrane attack complex (MAC). Ultrastructural studies reveal swollen damaged capillary endothelial cells containing undulating tubules or tubuloreticular structures.[21,24]

Most current models of muscle injury indicate that DM is a complement-mediated endomysial microvasculopathy.[14,25,26] Complement activation is thought to be an early pathologic feature preceding inflammation and myofiber injury. Activation of the complement C3 leads to formation of MAC, the lytic component of the complement pathway. MAC deposits on intramuscular capillaries and lyses capillary endothelial cells with subsequent vessel necrosis and perivascular inflammation. Progressive intramuscular vascular injury leads to capillary depletion and myofiber hypoperfusion and ischemia. The fibers at the peripheral watershed region of the fascicle, where there is normally a reduced capillary density, are more sensitive to the microvascular insults.[6] Cytokines and chemokines related to complement activation facilitate inflammatory cell recruitment to the perimysial and endomysial spaces.[14,27] Although the exact mechanisms of complement activation are unknown, many have implicated, but have not yet identified, autoantibodies directed against vascular endothelial antigens. Other suggested models of DM indicate that plasmacytoid dendritic cells overproduce interferons, leading to overexpression of intracellular proteins that mediate capillary injury and perifascicular myofiber atrophy.[11,23]

PM

PM is a disease of adults and shares many clinical features with DM. Patients with PM present with symmetric proximal muscle weakness usually more severe in the lower extremities than in the upper extremities. The weakness is progressive and develops over weeks to months. PM may also show extramuscular systemic manifestations, including interstitial lung disease, dysphagia, arthalgias, and cardiac arrhythmias. PM can be associated with various autoimmune diseases such as rheumatoid arthritis, lupus, or Sjögren syndrome.[14] Similar to DM, PM is also associated with an increased risk of malignancy.[15,16] The most important clinical finding that distinguishes PM from DM is the absence of the heliotrope rash, Gottron papules, and other cutaneous manifestations. Laboratory studies reveal that serum CK levels can be elevated up to 50-fold,[17] and various autoantibodies may also be seen.[14,26]

The myopathologic features that distinguish PM from DM are the absence of perifascicular atrophy and the presence of a multifocal endomysial inflammatory infiltrate composed primarily of lymphocytes and occasionally macrophages. The lymphocytes are CD8+ cytotoxic T suppressor cells that surround and invade intact, nonnecrotic, and morphologically normal-appearing myofibers (**Fig. 5**).[28] Immunohistochemical studies reveal that all myofibers (ie, those with and without lymphocytic invasion), show an increased expression of sarcolemmal MHC class I[22] that persists even after

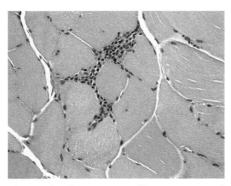

Fig. 5. Polymyositis. Endomysial inflammatory infiltrate composed of T lymphocytes surrounds and focally invades intact nonnecrotic myofibers (H&E, original magnification ×200).

administration of steroids.[29] The diffuse MHC class I overexpression in PM differs from that in DM, which is confined to damaged perifascicular muscle fibers. Other nonspecific findings such as variation in muscle fiber size, increased number of internalized myonuclei, scattered myofiber necrosis and regeneration, and fibrosis may be present. EM confirms the histologic findings and does not reveal any specific ultrastructural markers for PM.

PM is traditionally viewed as a cell-mediated autoimmune process with a clonal population of autoaggressive CD8+ T cells that invade nonnecrotic muscle fibers overexpressing MCH class I. Normal muscle fibers do not express MHC class I. However, muscle in patients with PM shows widespread MHC class I overexpression,[22] an early pathogenic feature that even precedes the inflammatory infiltrate.[30] It is thought that MHC class I molecules act as antigen-presenting cells to autoaggressive clonal T cells.[8] The T cells contain and release perforin and granulysin that induce myofiber lysis and necrosis.[31,32] Upregulation of numerous cytokines including interleukins, tumor necrosis factor α, and interferon γ may not only have direct myocytotoxic effects but also promote chronic inflammation and fibrosis.[14] Systemic retroviral infection has also been proposed to play a role in pathogenesis.[33]

sIBM

sIBM is an inflammatory myopathy of patients older than 40 years and is the most common IIM presenting in adults older than 50 years. sIBM presents with an insidious onset of proximal, lower extremity weakness that develops over months to years. Unlike in DM and PM, the weakness in sIBM can be asymmetric, more frequently involves the upper extremities, and involves distal muscle groups such as those of the wrist and forearms. At least 40% of patients may complain of dysphagia secondary to involvement of esophageal and pharyngeal muscles.[34] In contrast to DM and PM, interstitial lung disease in sIBM is rare and there is no association with myocarditis. Physical examination reveals a characteristic pattern of muscle atrophy involving the quadriceps and forearm flexor muscles. The serum CK level is frequently normal or only mildly elevated (<10-fold).[17]

Similar to PM, sIBM is characterized by a prominent endomysial inflammatory infiltrate of CD8+ lymphocytes and macrophages between and around muscle fibers (**Fig. 6**A). Lymphocytes, at least focally, invade intact nonnecrotic myofibers. The pathologic feature that distinguishes sIBM from PM on routine light microscopy is the presence of irregularly shaped vacuoles within myofibers. Typically, the vacuolated fibers are not invaded by lymphocytes.[6] Often the vacuoles appear empty, but

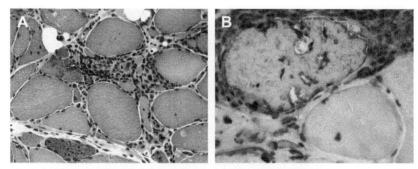

Fig. 6. Sporadic inclusion body myositis. (*A*) Intense endomysial inflammatory infiltrate, variation in fiber size and shape, and scattered fibers with vacuoles containing granular material (H&E, original magnification ×200). (*B*) Antibodies against SMI-31 highlight squiggly aggregates in the cytoplasm and around the rimmed vacuoles within an abnormal muscle fiber (original magnification ×400).

some are lined by granular material (rimmed vacuoles) that is basophilic on H&E stain and red on Gomori trichrome stain. Myonuclei in IBM are enlarged and morphologically abnormal, with disrupted nuclear membranes,[35] and rimmed vacuoles occasionally contain myonuclei.[34] Studies have shown that rimmed vacuoles are lined by nuclear proteins (eg, emerin and lamin A/C) and are thought to be possibly derived from myonuclei breakdown and/or are autophagic with abnormal lysosomal functions.[35,36] Ultrastructural studies reveal that vacuoles consist of multilaminated membranous structures; glycogen granules; dense bodies; and amorphous, granular, and fibrillar material.[37] Although thought to be a distinguishing feature of sIBM, rimmed vacuoles are occasionally seen in PM,[38] DM,[25] and distal myopathies, later-onset type II glycogenosis, myofibrillar myopathies, oculopharyngeal muscular dystrophy, and denervated muscle.[7,39]

Various multiprotein inclusion bodies may also be seen within myofibers.[40] Round plaquelike amyloid eosinophilic inclusions can be found in the cytoplasm or nucleus of vacuolated myofibers. These inclusions can be visualized with a Congo red stain with polarized light as apple green birefringence or with Texas red fluorescence microscopy. The congophilic inclusions immunoreact with various related proteins, including ubiquitin, β-amyloid, and β-amyloid precursor protein among others.[41] EM reveals amyloidlike fibrils that are 6 to 10 nm in diameter and are located in the cytoplasm.

A second type of myofiber inclusion, also congophilic,[42] is recognized with immunostaining with SMI-31 antibodies that highlight linear squiggly aggregates and aggregates around/near rimmed vacuoles (see **Fig. 6**B).[40] Antibodies for SMI-31 recognize several proteins including neurofilaments, phosphorylated tau, microtubule-associated proteins 1B and 2, lamin intermediate filament, and possibly sequestosome 1.[43] Although specific proteins recognized by SMI-31 antibodies in sIBM are unknown, many speculate that these inclusions represent abnormal aggregates of tau.[44] Ultrastructural studies reveal that these inclusions correspond to clusters of filaments 15 to 21 nm in diameter that resemble accumulations of tau paired helical filaments in Alzheimer disease.[40]

Recent studies have found abnormal accumulations of TAR DNA-binding protein (TDP)-43 in myofibers of sIBM.[45–48] TDP-43 is a nucleic acid–binding protein normally found within myocyte nuclei. In sIBM muscle, TDP-43 redistributes from myonuclei into the sarcoplasm forming punctate inclusions.[45,47] TDP-43 inclusions may contain ubiquitin[47] but do not appear to colocalize with SMI-31 or congophilic material.[39]

Redistribution of TDP-43 occurs much more frequently than other histologic markers of inclusion body myositis (IBM) (rimmed vacuoles, congophilic material, SMI-31 inclusions) and is a highly sensitive and specific feature for IBM.[45] Although the exact role that TDP-43 plays in IBM in unknown, TDP-43 could potentially be a standard diagnostic marker for sIBM.[49]

The precise cause of sIBM is unknown. Similar to PM, sIBM is characterized by MCH class I–restricted CD8+ T cell endomysial inflammation. However, unlike the other IIMs, sIBM does not respond to anti-inflammatory drugs, suggesting that IBM is a multifactorial myopathy with both inflammatory and noninflammatory components. In addition to tau, amyloid, and TDP-43, discussed earlier, there are accumulations of proteins αβ-crystallin,[50] apolipoprotein E,[44] presenilin 1,[51] and α-synuclein.[52] These proteins are linked to various neurodegenerative diseases, suggesting that sIBM could be a myodegenerative process. Similar to other neurodegenerative disorders, accumulations of unfolded and misfolded multiprotein complexes likely contributes to the pathogenesis of IBM.[40,53–55] In addition, abnormal accumulation of nitric oxide synthase and cellular protective enzymes (eg, superoxide dismutase) indicates an intracellular oxidative stress component, and the identification of ragged red and COX-negative fibers implicates mitochondrial abnormalities.[40]

In a patient with clinical features of IBM, the diagnosis is confirmed by characteristic features on muscle biopsy (ie, rimmed vacuoles, SMI staining, congophilic inclusions, tubulofilaments on EM). Many characteristics of IBM may be difficult to identify or are absent in an affected muscle on initial muscle biopsy because of sampling error, and the results of these biopsies frequently provide a diagnosis of PM.[56,57] Thus, when a clinician is confronted with a patient with PM refractory to immunosuppressive therapies or a patient with clinically suspected IBM with a prior biopsy suggesting PM, repeat muscle biopsies may be required for a definitive diagnosis.

DRUG-INDUCED MYOPATHIES

Numerous drugs and toxins can cause a myopathy. A drug- or toxin-induced myopathy should be clinically suspected in a patient who develops myopathic symptoms temporally related to the administration of a drug or exposure to a myotoxic substance. Clinical manifestations are typically nonspecific and include fatigue, muscle weakness, myalgia, elevated serum CK levels, myoglobinuria, and, rarely, rhabdomyolysis. Patients at higher risk of developing a drug- or toxin-induced myopathy are those with a decreased ability to metabolize or excrete the offending agent and/or its metabolites and include patients with liver failure, renal failure, infants and children, and the elderly.[3] There are many pathogenic mechanisms by which toxins and drugs cause muscle dysfunction. The types of abnormalities seen on muscle biopsy vary from nonspecific myopathic changes to specific and characteristic histopathologic findings. In this section, the authors highlight the pathologic findings of select drugs that have the potential to induce muscle toxicity and are commonly encountered by a clinical rheumatologist. This review is not all inclusive because these drugs as well as many other drugs and toxins have been extensively reviewed elsewhere.[3,4,58]

Statin-Induced Myopathy

The 3-hydroxy-3-methylglutaryl-CoA (HMGCoA) - reductase inhibitors (statins) are a dominant class of lipid-lowering drugs used in the treatment of hypercholesterolemia. Statin-induced myopathy presents with myalgia, weakness that is frequently symmetric involving proximal muscles, cramping, mild elevations in serum CK levels, and, rarely, rhabdomyolysis.[59,60] Patients can develop muscle symptoms during statin therapy or even months after the discontinuation of the offending agent. Several drugs can potentiate statin-induced myopathy and increase the incidence of rhabdomyolysis including other cholesterol-lowering agents (fibric acids and niacin), cyclosporine, erythromycin, warfarin, digoxin, diltiazem, and many others.[59–62] Many of these interactions are attributed to drug metabolism by cytochrome P450 system, especially those mediated through the cytochrome P450 3A4 isoenzyme pathway. In most patients, myopathic symptoms associated with statin therapy resolve within a few weeks after drug cessation. However, in a distinct immune-mediated subtype, myopathic symptoms do not improve after drug discontinuation and patients may require treatment with immunosuppressive agents.[63]

Muscle biopsy frequently reveals a necrotizing myopathy with myofiber necrosis and dissolution and invasion by macrophages (**Fig. 7**). Rarely, there is type II muscle fiber atrophy.[64] Increased lipid stores on oil red O stain, COX-negative fibers, and ragged red fibers on Gomori trichrome stain suggest mitochondrial dysfunction.[65] Lymphocytic infiltrate within nonnecrotic fibers, as can be seen in the IIMs (discussed earlier), is not prominent. EM confirms the light microscopic findings.

Although the exact molecular mechanisms of statin-induced myopathy are unknown, several hypotheses have been proposed and discussed in detail elsewhere.[59–62] Statins inhibit the enzyme HMGCoA reductase, the rate-limiting enzyme in cholesterol synthesis that converts HMGCoA to mevalonic acid. One hypothesis suggests that inhibition of HMGCoA reductase reduces cholesterol content in muscle membranes. Decreased cholesterol in sarcolemmal and mitochondrial membranes renders these membranes unstable with impaired membrane function and abnormal calcium influx. Other proposed theories focus on impaired synthesis of mevalonate. Mevalonate is the immediate precursors to isoprenoids in the cholesterol biosynthetic pathway. Isoprenoids are required for posttranslational lipid modification (prenylation) of numerous proteins. With statin therapy, reduced levels of isoprenoids and prenylated proteins result in impaired synthesis of tRNA, glycoproteins, and components of the electron transport chain including ubiquinone. Decreased prenylation of intracellular regulatory proteins, such as small GTP-binding proteins, are also thought to enhance apoptosis.

D-Penicillamine

D-Penicillamine is a degradation product of penicillin that chelates copper and other various metals. It is used in the treatment of Wilson disease, cystinuria, rheumatoid

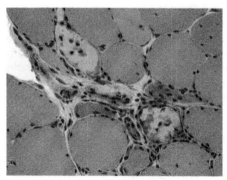

Fig. 7. Statin-induced myopathy. Necrotizing myopathy characterized by infiltration of macrophages and myofiber dissolution and necrosis (H&E, original magnification ×200).

arthritis, and various connective tissue disorders. D-Penicillamine is associated with an inflammatory myopathy that is clinically and histologically similar to idiopathic DM or PM. Patients can present at any time during the course of treatment with proximal muscle weakness and myalgia. Rare cases of fatal myocarditis secondary to cardiac involvement have been described.[66] Myopathic features of D-penicillamine–induced myopathy are histologically identical to those seen in DM or PM (see earlier discussion).[67]

D-Penicillamine is also reported to induce myasthenia gravis. Myasthenia gravis is associated with the production of autoantibodies directed at the acetylcholine receptor (AchR) or muscle-specific tyrosine kinase inhibitor (MuSK) at the neuromuscular junction. Diagnosis is typically made by a combination of clinical findings, serum AchR or MuSK autoantibodies, and pharmacologic and electrophysiologic tests. Typically, muscle biopsies are only performed to exclude other diagnoses and can show fiber atrophy, particularly type II fibers, with fiber type grouping, lymphoid aggregates (lymphorrhages), and COX-negative fibers and subsarcolemmal rims of mitochondria suggesting mitochondrial abnormalities.

AZT

AZT (3'-azido-2',3'-dideoxythymidine) is a nucleoside reverse transcriptase inhibitor used in the treatment of AIDS. The clinical features of AZT myopathy are similar to other human immunodeficiency virus (HIV)-associated myopathies (eg, HIV-associated PM) and include progressive proximal muscle weakness especially of lower extremities, myalgia, fatigue, and mildly elevated serum CK levels.[3] Myopathic symptoms typically develop after 6 to 12 months of treatment.[58] Muscle biopsy in AZT myopathy reveals features of a mitochondrial abnormality, including vacuolization, ragged red fibers on modified Gomori trichrome stain, and COX-negative fibers.[3,4] Pure AZT myopathy is not associated with a prominent endomysial inflammation that characterizes HIV-associated PM. EM reveals subsarcolemmal proliferations of abnormal mitochondria of various sizes and shapes with disorganized cristae.[68] AZT myopathy thought to result, in part, from AZT-mediated inhibition of mitochondrial γ-DNA polymerase, which is necessary for mitochondrial DNA replication.[69]

Colchicine

Colchicine is an alkaloid derivative derived from the plant *Colchicum autumale* used not only in the management of gout but also in the treatment of familial Mediterranean fever, Behçet disease, and other diseases.[70,71] Colchicine exerts it therapeutic effects by binding to β-tubulin monomers and preventing polymerization of tubulin into microtubules. Disruption of microtubule formation inhibits numerous intracellular processes, including mitosis.[72–74] Anti-inflammatory properties of colchicine are attributed, at least in part, to disrupted microtubule assembly in leukocytes resulting in altered adhesion, mobility, and cytokine production.[70,72]

Colchicine toxicity causes both a myopathy and a peripheral neuropathy. Most patients with colchicine-induced neuromyopathy present with progressive proximal muscle weakness and myalgia and rarely have mild sensory loss.[75] The serum CK level is typically elevated. Symptoms can present after acute intoxication or after chronic use and occurs more frequently in those with impaired renal function.[3]

On muscle biopsy, colchicine-induced toxicity causes a vacuolar myopathy. Within the cytoplasm of myocytes are variously sized vacuoles that may be empty or contain granular material (**Fig. 8**).[76] Within the vacuoles are accumulations of lysosomes and autophagic vacuoles that are thought to be derived from disruption of the cytoskeletal network.[75] Histochemical staining reveals that vacuoles are selective for type I fibers

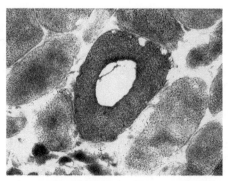

Fig. 8. Colchicine-induced myopathy. Variation in fiber size and shape and a single myofiber containing a central large vacuole and several small peripheral subsarcolemmal vacuoles. (NADH) (original magnification ×400).

and may stain for acid phosphatase. NADH staining shows foci of myofibrillar disorganization.[76] Prominent myonecrosis and inflammation is absent. Ultrastructural studies reveal autophagic vacuoles with whorled membranous and spheromembranous bodies.[21,77] Concomitant nerve biopsy may reveal a mild axonal neuropathy with loss of large myelinated axons.[75] A prominent neuropathic component may result in acute and/or chronic denervation myopathy characterized by angulated esterase-positive muscle fibers and/or fiber type grouping on muscle biopsy, respectively.

The myoneuropathy of colchicine toxicity is thought to result from disrupted microtubule networks that impair intracellular transport and accumulation of lysosomes with overproduction of autophagic vacuoles.[78,79]

Chloroquine and Hydroxychloroquine

Chloroquine and hydroxychloroquine are amphiphilic quinolones used in the treatment of malaria and various autoimmune disorders such as rheumatoid arthritis, systemic lupus erythematosus, sarcoidosis, and rheumatoid arthritis. Both drugs are associated with both a neuropathy and a polyneuropathy, although the neuromyotoxicity associated with chloroquine is more severe than that associated with hydroxychloroquine. Patients present with symmetric painless muscle weakness that begins in the proximal lower extremities and can slowly progress to involve the upper extremities and facial muscles. The polyneuropathy is characterized by decreased vibratory sensation and areflexia.[80] A restrictive cardiomyopathy with congestive heart failure can develop in some patients.[81] The serum CK level is often normal or mildly elevated. Neuromyotoxic symptoms typically develop months to years after the initiation of treatment and do not appear to be dose dependent.[80]

In chloroquine myopathy, muscle biopsy reveals myopathic changes with vacuolar degeneration. The vacuoles are present in approximately 50% of the myofibers and are preferentially located in type I fibers.[80] Histochemical staining reveals increased lysosomal enzyme activity with acid phosphatase stain.[82] Neurogenic muscle atrophy (angulated atrophic fibers, fiber type grouping) can also be seen. EM reveals sarcoplasmic degeneration products, such as curvilinear and membrane-bound concentric lamellar structures, called myeloid bodies (myelin figures) within vacuoles.[77,80] The findings on muscle biopsy in hydroxychloroquine toxicity are similar to those in chloroquine toxicity but are less severe with minimal to absent vacuolar changes. Endomyocardial muscle biopsies show changes similar to those in skeletal muscle.[83]

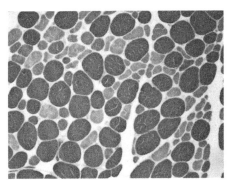

Fig. 9. Steroid-induced myopathy. Myofibrillary ATPase stain shows relative preservation of the darkly stained type I myofibers and selective atrophy of the lighter-stained type II myofibers (original magnification ×100).

Nerve biopsy shows demyelinization and degeneration of axons with accumulation of curvilinear and myeloid bodies.[82]

The mechanism of chloroquine and hydroxychloroquine myopathy is thought to be secondary to drug accumulation in lysosomes inhibiting various intralysosomal enzymes and protein degradation.

Corticosteroids

Patients exposed to corticosteroids can develop a steroid-induced myopathy. The source of corticosteroids can be endogenous hyperadrenocorticism (Cushing syndrome) or exogenous corticosteroid therapy. Fluorinated glucocorticoids (triamcinolone, betamethasone, and dexamethasone) may be more toxic than the nonfluorinated ones (prednisone, hydrocortisone).[84] There are 2 clinical patterns of myopathies attributed to steroids.[85] The classic presentation is a chronic steroid myopathy that develops after prolonged corticosteroid exposure. Patients complain of mild, slowly progressive, painless muscle weakness of the proximal part of upper and lower extremities. The serum CK level is normal or is only mildly elevated. The second presentation is an acute steroid myopathy and occurs less frequently than chronic steroid myopathy. Various terms have been used to describe this myopathy including acute quadriplegic myopathy and critical illness myopathy.[3] In acute steroid myopathy, patients develop severe generalized muscle weakness, some with complete flaccid paralysis, following short-term high-dose corticosteroid use. Muscle atrophy out of proportion for the degree of immobilization can occur.[86] Patients are frequently on mechanical ventilatory support, have asthmatic disorders, and receive neuromuscular blocking agents. The symptoms usually occur 5 to 7 days after initiation of steroids. The serum CK level is typically elevated, and myoglobinuria may be present.

In classical chronic steroid myopathy, muscle biopsy shows selective atrophy of type II fibers (**Fig. 9**), especially fast twitch type IIB glycolytic fibers,[85] identified with ATPase and NADH enzyme histochemical stains. There is no significant inflammation or necrosis. Ultrastructural analysis may reveal mild mitochondrial abnormalities.[3] In acute steroid myopathy, muscle biopsy reveals atrophy of type II myofibers, with or without type I myofiber atrophy, with focal or diffuse necrosis.[3,85] EM reveals selective loss of myosin thick filaments.[3]

The exact mechanism of steroid myopathy is unknown but is speculated to be multifactorial, involving alterations in protein synthesis and degradation, abnormal carbohydrate metabolism with glycogen accumulation, altered mitochondria, acquired channelopathies, and many others.[3,86–88]

SUMMARY

The pathologic workup for muscle biopsies is one of the most complex, extensive, and expensive procedures because of the numerous types of specimen processing, staining, and histologic, ultrastructural, biochemical, and genetic studies needed to render a diagnosis. Despite the extensive workup of muscle biopsies, neuropathologists cannot always define a specific cause of the muscle pathology and rely on a close working relationship with the clinical team to come up with a clinical-pathologic working diagnosis.

REFERENCES

1. Kuo GP, Carrino JA. Skeletal muscle imaging and inflammatory myopathies. Curr Opin Rheumatol 2007;19(6):530–5.
2. Rahman S, Hanna MG. Diagnosis and therapy in neuromuscular disorders: diagnosis and new treatments in mitochondrial diseases. J Neurol Neurosurg Psychiatry 2009;80(9):943–53.
3. Walsh RJ, Amato AA. Toxic myopathies. Neurol Clin 2005;23(2):397–428.
4. Guis S, Mattei JP, Liote F. Drug-induced and toxic myopathies. Best Pract Res Clin Rheumatol 2003;17(6):877–907.
5. van Adel BA, Tarnopolsky MA. Metabolic myopathies: update 2009. J Clin Neuromuscul Dis 2009;10(3):97–121.
6. Dalakas MC. Muscle biopsy findings in inflammatory myopathies. Rheum Dis Clin North Am 2002;28(4):779–98, vi.
7. Hewer E, Goebel HH. Myopathology of non-infectious inflammatory myopathies - the current status. Pathol Res Pract 2008;204(9):609–23.
8. Dalakas MC. Mechanisms of disease: signaling pathways and immunobiology of inflammatory myopathies. Nat Clin Pract Rheumatol 2006;2(4):219–27.
9. Greenberg SA. Inflammatory myopathies: disease mechanisms. Curr Opin Neurol 2009;22(5):516–23.
10. Dalakas MC. Inflammatory disorders of muscle: progress in polymyositis, dermatomyositis and inclusion body myositis. Curr Opin Neurol 2004;17(5):561–7.
11. Greenberg SA. Proposed immunologic models of the inflammatory myopathies and potential therapeutic implications. Neurology 2007;69(21):2008–19.
12. Amato AA, Barohn RJ. Evaluation and treatment of inflammatory myopathies. J Neurol Neurosurg Psychiatry 2009;80(10):1060–8.
13. Callen JP, Wortmann RL. Dermatomyositis. Clin Dermatol 2006;24(5):363–73.
14. Dalakas MC, Hohlfeld R. Polymyositis and dermatomyositis. Lancet 2003; 362(9388):971–82.
15. Buchbinder R, Hill CL. Malignancy in patients with inflammatory myopathy. Curr Rheumatol Rep 2002;4(5):415–26.
16. Hill CL, Zhang Y, Sigurgeirsson B, et al. Frequency of specific cancer types in dermatomyositis and polymyositis: a population-based study. Lancet 2001; 357(9250):96–100.
17. Wiendl H. Idiopathic inflammatory myopathies: current and future therapeutic options. Neurotherapeutics 2008;5(4):548–57.
18. Targoff IN. Laboratory testing in the diagnosis and management of idiopathic inflammatory myopathies. Rheum Dis Clin North Am 2002;28(4):859–90, viii.

19. Gunawardena H, Betteridge ZE, McHugh NJ. Myositis-specific autoantibodies: their clinical and pathogenic significance in disease expression. Rheumatology (Oxford) 2009;48(6):607–12.
20. Limaye VS, Blumbergs P, Roberts-Thomson PJ. Idiopathic inflammatory myopathies. Intern Med J 2009;39(3):179–90.
21. Lane R. Toxic and drug-induced myopathies. In: Houston MJ, Cook L, editors. Muscle biopsy a practical approach. 3rd edition. Philadelphia/Amsterdam: Saunders/Elsevier; 2007. p. 541–55.
22. Karpati G, Pouliot Y, Carpenter S. Expression of immunoreactive major histocompatibility complex products in human skeletal muscles. Ann Neurol 1988;23(1): 64–72.
23. Greenberg SA, Pinkus JL, Pinkus GS, et al. Interferon-alpha/beta-mediated innate immune mechanisms in dermatomyositis. Ann Neurol 2005;57(5):664–78.
24. De Visser M, Emslie-Smith AM, Engel AG. Early ultrastructural alterations in adult dermatomyositis. Capillary abnormalities precede other structural changes in muscle. J Neurol Sci 1989;94(1–3):181–92.
25. Limaye VS, Blumbergs P. The prevalence of rimmed vacuoles in biopsy-proven dermatomyositis. Muscle Nerve 2010;41(2):288–9; 288.
26. Mammen AL. Dermatomyositis and polymyositis: clinical presentation, autoantibodies, and pathogenesis. Ann N Y Acad Sci 2010;1184:134–53.
27. De Paepe B, Creus KK, De Bleecker JL. Role of cytokines and chemokines in idiopathic inflammatory myopathies. Curr Opin Rheumatol 2009;21(6):610–6.
28. Arahata K, Engel AG. Monoclonal antibody analysis of mononuclear cells in myopathies. I: quantitation of subsets according to diagnosis and sites of accumulation and demonstration and counts of muscle fibers invaded by T cells. Ann Neurol 1984;16(2):193–208.
29. Nyberg P, Wikman AL, Nennesmo I, et al. Increased expression of interleukin 1alpha and MHC class I in muscle tissue of patients with chronic, inactive polymyositis and dermatomyositis. J Rheumatol 2000;27(4):940–8.
30. Tajima Y, Moriwaka F, Tashiro K. Temporal alterations of immunohistochemical findings in polymyositis. Intern Med 1994;33(5):263–70.
31. Goebels N, Michaelis D, Engelhardt M, et al. Differential expression of perforin in muscle-infiltrating T cells in polymyositis and dermatomyositis. J Clin Invest 1996; 97(12):2905–10.
32. Ikezoe K, Ohshima S, Osoegawa M, et al. Expression of granulysin in polymyositis and inclusion-body myositis. J Neurol Neurosurg Psychiatry 2006;77(10):1187–90.
33. Dalakas MC. Inflammatory, immune, and viral aspects of inclusion-body myositis. Neurology 2006;66(2 Suppl 1):S33–8.
34. Amato AA, Barohn RJ. Inclusion body myositis: old and new concepts. J Neurol Neurosurg Psychiatry 2009;80(11):1186–93.
35. Greenberg SA, Pinkus JL, Amato AA. Nuclear membrane proteins are present within rimmed vacuoles in inclusion-body myositis. Muscle Nerve 2006;34(4): 406–16.
36. Kumamoto T, Ueyama H, Tsumura H, et al. Expression of lysosome-related proteins and genes in the skeletal muscles of inclusion body myositis. Acta Neuropathol 2004;107(1):59–65.
37. Fukuhara N, Kumamoto T, Tsubaki T. Rimmed vacuoles. Acta Neuropathol 1980; 51(3):229–35.
38. van der Meulen MF, Hoogendijk JE, Moons KG, et al. Rimmed vacuoles and the added value of SMI-31 staining in diagnosing sporadic inclusion body myositis. Neuromuscul Disord 2001;11(5):447–51.

39. Schoser B. Physiology, pathophysiology and diagnostic significance of autophagic changes in skeletal muscle tissue–towards the enigma of rimmed and round vacuoles. Clin Neuropathol 2009;28(1):59–70.

40. Askanas V, Engel WK. Inclusion-body myositis: newest concepts of pathogenesis and relation to aging and Alzheimer disease. J Neuropathol Exp Neurol 2001; 60(1):1–14.

41. Askanas V, Engel WK, Bilak M, et al. Twisted tubulofilaments of inclusion body myositis muscle resemble paired helical filaments of Alzheimer brain and contain hyperphosphorylated tau. Am J Pathol 1994;144(1):177–87.

42. Mirabella M, Alvarez RB, Engel WK, et al. Apolipoprotein E and apolipoprotein E messenger RNA in muscle of inclusion body myositis and myopathies. Ann Neurol 1996;40(6):864–72.

43. Salajegheh M, Pinkus JL, Nazareno R, et al. Nature of "Tau" immunoreactivity in normal myonuclei and inclusion body myositis. Muscle Nerve 2009;40(4): 520–8.

44. Mirabella M, Alvarez RB, Bilak M, et al. Difference in expression of phosphorylated tau epitopes between sporadic inclusion-body myositis and hereditary inclusion-body myopathies. J Neuropathol Exp Neurol 1996;55(7):774–86.

45. Salajegheh M, Pinkus JL, Taylor JP, et al. Sarcoplasmic redistribution of nuclear TDP-43 in inclusion body myositis. Muscle Nerve 2009;40(1):19–31.

46. Olive M, Janue A, Moreno D, et al. TAR DNA-Binding protein 43 accumulation in protein aggregate myopathies. J Neuropathol Exp Neurol 2009;68(3): 262–73.

47. Weihl CC, Temiz P, Miller SE, et al. TDP-43 accumulation in inclusion body myopathy muscle suggests a common pathogenic mechanism with frontotemporal dementia. J Neurol Neurosurg Psychiatry 2008;79(10):1186–9.

48. Kusters B, van Hoeve BJ, Schelhaas HJ, et al. TDP-43 accumulation is common in myopathies with rimmed vacuoles. Acta Neuropathol 2009;117(2):209–11.

49. Verma A, Tandan R. TDP-43: a reliable immunohistochemistry marker for inclusion body myositis? Muscle Nerve 2009;40(1):8–9.

50. Banwell BL, Engel AG. AlphaB-crystallin immunolocalization yields new insights into inclusion body myositis. Neurology 2000;54(5):1033–41.

51. Askanas V, Engel WK, Yang CC, et al. Light and electron microscopic immunolocalization of presenilin 1 in abnormal muscle fibers of patients with sporadic inclusion-body myositis and autosomal-recessive inclusion-body myopathy. Am J Pathol 1998;152(4):889–95.

52. Askanas V, Engel WK, Alvarez RB, et al. Novel immunolocalization of alpha-synuclein in human muscle of inclusion-body myositis, regenerating and necrotic muscle fibers, and at neuromuscular junctions. J Neuropathol Exp Neurol 2000; 59(7):592–8.

53. Askanas V, Engel WK. Proposed pathogenetic cascade of inclusion-body myositis: importance of amyloid-beta, misfolded proteins, predisposing genes, and aging. Curr Opin Rheumatol 2003;15(6):737–44.

54. Askanas V, Engel WK. Inclusion-body myositis, a multifactorial muscle disease associated with aging: current concepts of pathogenesis. Curr Opin Rheumatol 2007;19(6):550–9.

55. Askanas V, Engel WK. Inclusion-body myositis: a myodegenerative conformational disorder associated with Abeta, protein misfolding, and proteasome inhibition. Neurology 2006;66(2 Suppl 1):S39–48.

56. Amato AA, Gronseth GS, Jackson CE, et al. Inclusion body myositis: clinical and pathological boundaries. Ann Neurol 1996;40(4):581–6.

57. van der Meulen MF, Hoogendijk JE, Jansen GH, et al. Absence of characteristic features in two patients with inclusion body myositis. J Neurol Neurosurg Psychiatry 1998;64(3):396–8.

58. Dalakas MC. Toxic and drug-induced myopathies. J Neurol Neurosurg Psychiatry 2009;80(8):832–8.

59. Baer AN, Wortmann RL. Myotoxicity associated with lipid-lowering drugs. Curr Opin Rheumatol 2007;19(1):67–73.

60. Thompson PD, Clarkson P, Karas RH. Statin-associated myopathy. JAMA 2003; 289(13):1681–90.

61. Baker SK, Tarnopolsky MA. Statin myopathies: pathophysiologic and clinical perspectives. Clin Invest Med 2001;24(5):258–72.

62. Mukhtar RY, Reckless JP. Statin-induced myositis: a commonly encountered or rare side effect? Curr Opin Lipidol 2005;16(6):640–7.

63. Grable-Esposito P, Katzberg HD, Greenberg SA, et al. Immune-mediated necrotizing myopathy associated with statins. Muscle Nerve 2010;41(2):185–90.

64. Meriggioli MN, Barboi AC, Rowin J, et al. HMG-CoA reductase inhibitor myopathy: clinical, electrophysiological, and pathologic data in five patients. J Clin Neuromuscul Dis 2001;2(3):129–34.

65. Phillips PS, Haas RH, Bannykh S, et al. Statin-associated myopathy with normal creatine kinase levels. Ann Intern Med 2002;137(7):581–5.

66. Doyle DR, McCurley TL, Sergent JS. Fatal polymyositis in D-penicillamine-treated rheumatoid arthritis. Ann Intern Med 1983;98(3):327–30.

67. Petersen J, Halberg P, Hojgaard K, et al. Penicillamine-induced polymyositis-dermatomyositis. Scand J Rheumatol 1978;7(2):113–7.

68. Pezeshkpour G, Illa I, Dalakas MC. Ultrastructural characteristics and DNA immunocytochemistry in human immunodeficiency virus and zidovudine-associated myopathies. Hum Pathol 1991;22(12):1281–8.

69. Scruggs ER, Dirks Naylor AJ. Mechanisms of zidovudine-induced mitochondrial toxicity and myopathy. Pharmacology 2008;82(2):83–8.

70. Niel E, Scherrmann JM. Colchicine today. Joint Bone Spine 2006;73(6):672–8.

71. Bhat A, Naguwa SM, Cheema GS, et al. Colchicine revisited. Ann N Y Acad Sci 2009;1173:766–73.

72. Molad Y. Update on colchicine and its mechanism of action. Curr Rheumatol Rep 2002;4(3):252–6.

73. Ben-Chetrit E, Bergmann S, Sood R. Mechanism of the anti-inflammatory effect of colchicine in rheumatic diseases: a possible new outlook through microarray analysis. Rheumatology (Oxford) 2006;45(3):274–82.

74. Terkeltaub RA. Colchicine update: 2008. Semin Arthritis Rheum 2009;38(6):411–9.

75. Wilbur K, Makowsky M. Colchicine myotoxicity: case reports and literature review. Pharmacotherapy 2004;24(12):1784–92.

76. Fernandez C, Figarella-Branger D, Alla P, et al. Colchicine myopathy: a vacuolar myopathy with selective type I muscle fiber involvement. An immunohistochemical and electron microscopic study of two cases. Acta Neuropathol 2002; 103(2):100–6.

77. Lonesky TA, Kreuter JD, Wortmann RL, et al. Hydroxychloroquine and colchicine induced myopathy. J Rheumatol 2009;36(11):2617–8.

78. Kuncl RW. Agents and mechanisms of toxic myopathy. Curr Opin Neurol 2009; 22(5):506–15.

79. Kuncl RW, Bilak MM, Craig SW, et al. Exocytotic "constipation" is a mechanism of tubulin/lysosomal interaction in colchicine myopathy. Exp Cell Res 2003;285(2): 196–207.

80. Estes ML, Ewing-Wilson D, Chou SM, et al. Chloroquine neuromyotoxicity. Clinical and pathologic perspective. Am J Med 1987;82(3):447–55.
81. Iglesias Cubero G, Rodriguez Reguero JJ, Rojo Ortega JM. Restrictive cardiomyopathy caused by chloroquine. Br Heart J 1993;69(5):451–2.
82. Finsterer J, Jarius C. Increased CSF protein in chloroquine-induced axonal polyneuropathy and myopathy. Clin Neurol Neurosurg 2003;105(4):231–6.
83. Baguet JP, Tremel F, Fabre M. Chloroquine cardiomyopathy with conduction disorders. Heart 1999;81(2):221–3.
84. Faludi G, Gotlieb J, Meyers J. Factors influencing the development of steroid-induced myopathies. Ann N Y Acad Sci 1966;138(1):62–72.
85. Dekhuijzen PN, Decramer M. Steroid-induced myopathy and its significance to respiratory disease: a known disease rediscovered. Eur Respir J 1992;5(8):997–1003.
86. Zink W, Kollmar R, Schwab S. Critical illness polyneuropathy and myopathy in the intensive care unit. Nat Rev Neurol 2009;5(7):372–9.
87. Owczarek J, Jasinska M, Orszulak-Michalak D. Drug-induced myopathies. An overview of the possible mechanisms. Pharmacol Rep 2005;57(1):23–34.
88. Polsonetti BW, Joy SD, Laos LF. Steroid-induced myopathy in the ICU. Ann Pharmacother 2002;36(11):1741–4.

Index

Note: Page numbers of article titles are in **boldface** type.

A

Acid α-glucosidase deficiency (Pompe disease), 208, 237, 241, 293
Actin defects, in myopathies, 280
Acyl-coenzyme A dehydrogenase deficiency, 294
Adaptive devices, for muscular dystrophy, 242–243
Adaptive immune response, in polymyositis and dermatomyositis, 159–162
Aggregates, in inclusion body myositis, 298
Aldolase, in myositis, 151
Alemtuzumab, for inclusion body myositis, 179
Allele-specific oligonucleotide analysis, for myopathies, 274
Aminoacyl-transfer RNA synthetase, antibodies to, in polymyositis and dermatomyositis, 150, 160–161
Aminoglycoside-induced deafness, 281
Amiodarone, myopathy due to, 221–222
Amyloid deposits, in inclusion body myositis, 176–178, 298
Amyopathic dermatomyositis, 144, 147–148
Andersen disease (glycogen storage disease type IV), 208
Anesthetics, malignant hyperthermia due to, 225
Angina, in dermatomyositis, 149
Antiaminoacyl-transfer RNA synthetase antibodies, in polymyositis and dermatomyositis, 150, 160–161
Antiarrhythmic agents, myopathy due to, 221–222
Antibacterial agents, myopathy due to, 224
Antibodies. *See also specific antibodies.*
    in polymyositis and dermatomyositis, 150–152, 191
Antifungal agents, myopathy due to, 224
Antihistidyl-tRNA synthetase antibodies, in polymyositis and dermatomyositis, 150, 160
Antimicrobials, myopathy due to, 223–224
Antinuclear antibodies, in polymyositis and dermatomyositis, 160
Antipsychotics, myopathy due to, 225
Antisynthetase autoantibodies, 152
Anti-T-lymphocyte globulin, for inclusion body myositis, 179
Antiviral agents, myopathy due to, 223–224
Apoptosis, in polymyositis and dermatomyositis, 165–166
Arimoclomol, for inclusion body myositis, 179
Arrhythmias
    in dermatomyositis, 148–149
    in muscular dystrophy, 242
Arthralgia and arthritis, in polymyositis and dermatomyositis, 145
Aspiration pneumonia, in polymyositis and dermatomyositis, 149–150
Atorvastatin, myopathy due to, 219–221
Autoimmune necrotizing myopathy, 154–155

Rheum Dis Clin N Am 37 (2011) 309–322
doi:10.1016/S0889-857X(11)00021-4
0889-857X/11/$ – see front matter © 2011 Elsevier Inc. All rights reserved.
rheumatic.theclinics.com

Moving?

Make sure your subscription moves with you!

To notify us of your new address, find your **Clinics Account Number** (located on your mailing label above your name), and contact customer service at:

Email: journalscustomerservice-usa@elsevier.com

800-654-2452 (subscribers in the U.S. & Canada)
314-447-8871 (subscribers outside of the U.S. & Canada)

Fax number: 314-447-8029

Elsevier Health Sciences Division
Subscription Customer Service
3251 Riverport Lane
Maryland Heights, MO 63043

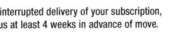

*To ensure uninterrupted delivery of your subscription, please notify us at least 4 weeks in advance of move.

ELSEVIER

Printed and bound by CPI Group (UK) Ltd, Croydon, CR0 4YY

03/10/2024

01040459-0020